THE EARLY DIAGNOSIS OF THE ACUTE ABDOMEN

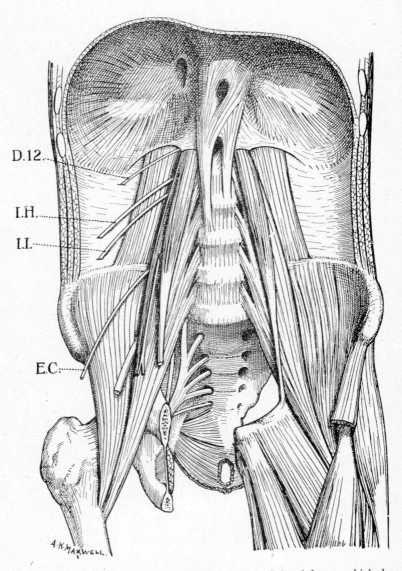

D.12

I.H.

I.I.

E.C.

Fig. 1.—Drawing to show the parietal muscles of the abdomen which, by their rigidity, immobility, and tenderness, give important help in diagnosis of the acute abdomen. (On the right side the twelfth dorsal nerve, and the ilio-hypogastric, ilio-inguinal, external cutaneous, and genito-crural nerves are indicated.)

[Frontispiece

OXFORD MEDICAL PUBLICATIONS

THE EARLY DIAGNOSIS
OF
THE ACUTE ABDOMEN

BY

ZACHARY COPE
B.A., M.D., M.S. Lond., F.R.C.S. Eng.

CONSULTING SURGEON TO ST. MARY'S HOSPITAL, PADDINGTON, AND TO THE BOLINGBROKE
HOSPITAL, WANDSWORTH COMMON; LATE HUNTERIAN PROFESSOR, ARRIS AND GALE AND
BRADSHAW LECTURER, ROYAL COLLEGE OF SURGEONS

TENTH EDITION

GEOFFREY CUMBERLEGE
OXFORD UNIVERSITY PRESS
LONDON   NEW YORK   TORONTO
1951

Oxford University Press, Amen House, London E.C.4

GLASGOW NEW YORK TORONTO MELBOURNE WELLINGTON
BOMBAY CALCUTTA MADRAS CAPE TOWN

Geoffrey Cumberlege, Publisher to the University

First Edition	1921
Second Edition	1923
Second Impression	1924
Third Edition	1925
Second Impression	1926
Fourth Edition	1927
Fifth Edition	1928
Second Impression	1930
Sixth Edition	1932
Seventh Edition	1935
Second Impression	1937
Eighth Edition	1940
Second Impression	1940
Third Impression	1942
Fourth Impression	1944
Ninth Edition	1946
Second Impression	1947
Third Impression	1948
Tenth Edition	1951

PRINTED IN GREAT BRITAIN BY
HAZELL WATSON AND VINEY LTD
AYLESBURY AND LONDON

PREFACE TO THE TENTH EDITION

No essential change has been made in this edition, but the opportunity has been taken to make some minor alterations and to add a few paragraphs to bring the teaching up-to-date. One additional radiograph has been inserted, for which I am indebted to Dr. Rohan Williams. The author hopes that the book may continue to help students and practitioners to diagnose this often difficult class of case.

ZACHARY COPE

London, N.W.3
January 1951

PREFACE TO THE NINTH EDITION

THE call for a ninth edition has enabled me to make a few minor alterations and additions, chiefly in Chapters VII and XI. I am grateful to Mr. Netley Scarle and Mr. Keith Vartan for useful hints, and to Mr. Courtney Gage for so kindly providing Figures 21 and 23.

During the War I have met many doctors from the United States of America and from all parts of the British Commonwealth who have generously expressed their indebtedness to this little book; I would like to take this opportunity of letting them know how much pleasure and encouragement their testimony gave me.

ZACHARY COPE

London, W.1
April 1945

PREFACE TO THE FIRST EDITION

ALL who have had much experience of the group of cases known generally as the acute abdomen will probably agree that in that condition early diagnosis is exceptional. There are still many who do not appreciate to the full the significance of the earlier and less flagrant symptoms of acute abdominal disease, who regard an increased frequency of the pulse and rigidity of the overlying abdominal muscles as necessary accompaniments of the early stage of appendicitis, or find it hard to believe that a patient with a non-distended abdomen and normal pulse and temperature can be the victim of a perforated gastric ulcer.

It would appear, therefore, that there is room for a small book dealing solely with the early diagnosis of such cases, for there is little need to labour the truism that earlier diagnosis means better prognosis. Though the present attempt to supply the deficiency may be inadequate, the author has at least endeavoured to assist the reader to attain a correct judgment in the evaluation of the various puzzling symptoms present in urgent abdominal disease.

Few references are inserted and no bibliography is appended ; for whilst the writer readily acknowledges the great debt which he owes to the teaching of such leaders as Murphy, Moynihan, Rutherford Morison, Maylard, and many others, it has been his aim to put down nothing which has not been frequently confirmed and demonstrated in his own experience.

At the same time he has introduced many diagnostic points which he believes have either never previously been recorded or to which insufficient attention is usually paid. In the former category may be mentioned the localizing diagnostic value of phrenic shoulder-pain, the obturator test, and the test for differentiating between pain of thoracic and abdominal origin; whilst in the latter the area of hyperæsthesia caused by a distended inflamed appendix, the pathognomonic axillary area of liver resonance in cases of perforated ulcer, the psoas-extension test, and the confusing significance of testicular pain, serve as examples.

ZACHARY COPE

LONDON
June 1921

CONTENTS

xi

CONTENTS

LIST OF ILLUSTRATIONS

LIST OF ILLUSTRATIONS

THE EARLY DIAGNOSIS OF THE ACUTE ABDOMEN

" There is surely no greater wisdom than well to time the beginning and onsets of things."—BACON, *Essay on " Delay."*

CHAPTER I

THE PRINCIPLES OF DIAGNOSIS IN ACUTE ABDOMINAL DISEASE

BEFORE entering on the detailed consideration of the methods of examination of the various forms of the acute abdomen, it is well to lay down certain principles which form the basis of all successful diagnosis in urgent abdominal disease.

1. The first principle is that of the *necessity of making a serious and thorough attempt at diagnosis.*

Abdominal pain is one of the most common conditions which call for speedy diagnosis and treatment. Usually, though by no means always, there are other symptoms which accompany the pain, but in the majority of cases of acute abdominal disease pain is the main symptom and complaint. The very terms " acute abdomen " and " abdominal emergency," which are constantly applied to such cases, signify the urgent need for prompt diagnosis and active treatment. It is common knowledge, however, that when confronted with a patient suffering great abdominal pain it is often very difficult to be certain as to the exact intra-abdominal lesion which has given rise to the symptoms.   In some instances the urgent need for surgical assistance may be so obvious that the need of transference of the patient to a surgical centre is clear.   In other cases the observer may, if in doubt, think it discreet to discuss the problem with a fellow-practitioner before deciding on any course of action. There are, however, occasions when, with some-what indefinite symptoms, there may be a tendency to wait for the development of clearer indications, to see if the condition will not improve spontaneously, and generally to temporize.   The last course of conduct is the least justifiable, for it is a wise plan always to make a very thorough attempt to elucidate the problem when the patient is seen for the first time.   Though in quite a number of cases it is impossible to be sure of the diagnosis, yet it is a good habit to come to a decision in each case ; and it will be found that after a short time, provided that no method of diagnosis be neglected, the percentage of correct diagnoses will rapidly increase.

That there is much room for improvement in this direction cannot be gainsaid.   Even the operating surgeon is not free from blame in this matter, for the ease and comparative safety of operating occasionally cause him to make a rather perfunctory examination of some patients whom from previous experience he judges to be in urgent need of abdominal section.   If every surgeon were to make an exhaustive attempt at a full diagnosis before operating, the science of elucidation of acute

abdominal disease would be advanced considerably.   There is no field in which diagnosis should
be so precise, since in no class of cases has the
surgeon so great an opportunity of correlating
the symptoms with the pathology of the living.

It is only by thorough examination that one can
propound a diagnosis, and if the early stages of the
disease are to be recognized note must be taken of
the earliest symptoms.   The general practitioners
have better opportunities than any other section
of the medical community for observing these early
symptoms, and by patient and painstaking observation it is possible for them greatly to add to
the stock of common knowledge.   To attempt a
diagnosis prevents carelessness, and carelessness in
urgent abdominal diagnosis is close akin to callous-
ness.

It is a truism to say that correct diagnosis
is the essential preliminary to correct treatment.
Many and serious results have followed from an
observer jumping to wrong conclusions which might
easily have been avoided by a real attempt at
clinical differentiation.

Spot-diagnosis may be magnificent, but it is not
sound diagnosis.   It is impressive but unsafe.   The
deduction and induction from observed facts necessary for the formation of a definite opinion are
good mental discipline for the observer, help to
imprint upon the tables of the mind perceptions
and clinical pictures which can usefully be recalled
in the future, and give a sense of satisfaction which
is only slightly diminished if the resulting opinion
should prove to be incorrect.   One often, if not
always, learns more by analysing the process of and

detecting the fallacy in an incorrect diagnosis than by taking unction to oneself when the diagnosis proves correct.

2. There can be no question that in acute abdominal disease it is of the utmost importance to *diagnose early.* Like the business man who takes as his motto "Do it now," the medical man, when confronted with an urgent abdominal case, should have ever before him the words "Diagnose now." The patient cries out for relief, the relatives are insistent that something shall be done, and the humane disciple of Æsculapius may think it his first duty to diminish or banish the too obvious agony by administering a narcotic. Such a policy is often literally a fatal mistake. Though it may appear cruel, it is really kind to withhold morphine until one is certain whether or not surgical interference is necessary, i.e. until a reasonable diagnosis has been made. Morphine does little or nothing to stop serious intra-abdominal disease, but it puts an efficient screen in front of the symptoms. The fire burns, but it is not visible, and sometimes only when vitality is burnt out is the mistake realized. If morphine be administered, it is possible for a patient to die happy in the belief that he is on the road to recovery, and in some cases the medical attendant may for a time be induced to share the delusive hope.

It is a curious but well-known fact that many who are taken with abdominal pain in the daytime endure till evening before they feel compelled to send for the doctor. It follows that important decisions often have to be made at night when the physician, weary with the day's work, and with perceptions and reasoning faculties somewhat jaded, is both physically and mentally below his best. The temptation is often very strong to temporize and " see how things are in the morning." There can be few practitioners of experience who cannot look back with regret to one or more occasions when delay has been fraught with disaster. The waiting attitude is understandable, but only occasionally excusable. To suspect an intussusception, to think that possibly there may be a perforation of a gastric ulcer, and yet to leave the question undecided for eight or ten hours, is to gamble with a life. A delay of two hours in diagnosis may make the difference between two weeks' and two months' illness of the patient. The fact that the patient comes late to the doctor is all the greater reason why he should diagnose as soon as possible. *The general rule can be laid down that the majority of severe abdominal pains which ensue in patients who have been previously fairly well, and which last as long as six hours, are caused by conditions of surgical import.* There are exceptions, but the generalization is useful if it serves to call attention to the need for early diagnosis. It is now acknowledged by those who are acquainted with modern surgical results that the best treatment for perforated ulcers, appendicitis, ectopic gestation, and intestinal obstruction is by surgical intervention. It is also well recognized that the earlier such cases come to the surgeon the better are the results. When it is remembered, however, that the first successful suture of a perforated gastric ulcer was performed less than sixty years ago, that the removal of a diseased appendix has only been a practical surgical question for about the same time, that opening the abdomen for intestinal obstruction was regarded at the beginning of this century as the last instead of the first resort, it will be recognized that the modern mental attitude toward abdominal emergencies has only been adopted within the lifetime of this generation. But the old view that delay is permissible still lingers in some quarters, for custom changes slowly. Public opinion on the subject needs education, and such education must come from the practitioner. The attitude of some patients who assert—and act up to their assertion—that they would rather die without operation than obtain a good chance of cure by undergoing some surgical procedure, is surely the result of an imperfect diffusion of the knowledge that surgery offers the best chance of life in such emergencies.

The recovery-rate from acute abdominal disease increases in proportion to the earliness of diagnosis and treatment. For the first time since this book was written we are able to report a considerable reduction in the mortality from acute abdominal disease in England and Wales, particularly in the case of the infective processes. In the decade 1938–48 the annual number of deaths from appendicitis dropped from 3,027 to 1,257, while a similar reduction in mortality occurred with cholecystitis. This great improvement may have been due to several causes— the introduction of the antibiotics, the increase in the number of trained surgeons, or even the diminution of the amount of meat eaten—but we believe it possible or even likely that some of the improvement may be due to earlier diagnosis. This view is supported by the fact that during the same ten years

the annual mortality from ectopic gestation dropped
from 75 to 34, for early diagnosis is of great importance in the prognosis of this condition.

But during this same ten years the number of
deaths from intestinal obstruction did not decrease
in quite so great a proportion and in the case of
hernia the reduction was still less—1,925 deaths
in 1938, 1,746 in 1948. Though we are furnished
with no particulars, it is clear that most of
these herniæ must have been obstructed or
strangulated. A strangulated hernia is that form
of intestinal obstruction which should be, and most
probably is, most readily diagnosed. Why, then,
the mortality? Because it is not realized that
the dangers of prompt operative interference are
less than those of waiting and seeing if the accompanying obstruction will right itself under
treatment of a non-operative character. Fomentations and icebags are not so safe as a knife and
a few sutures. Taxis is in the writer's view only
justifiable when dealing with an *easily* reducible
hernia.

If, in cases showing such an obvious cause for
intestinal obstruction as a strangulated hernia,
delay is permitted, we can the more readily understand how the remaining statistics mentioned above
are produced. In early diagnosis lies the saving of
thousands of lives.

3. The necessity of the principle of making a
thorough routine examination of every acute abdominal case should not need much emphasis. If one
is to make a correct diagnosis a complete routine
examination should be the rule. Few omit to
feel the pulse and take the temperature—yet

many a serious abdominal crisis may show at the time of examination a normal pulse and temperature. It is more important to insert the finger into the lower end than to put the thermometer into the upper end of the alimentary tract. More early cases will be diagnosed by palpating the pelvic peritoneum than by palpating the pulse. Few would forget to ask whether the bowels were constipated or not, but many might forget that it is quite as important to submit the urine to the chemical question of boiling. In the most perfunctory examination one is almost bound to lay the hand on the patient's abdomen, and if the latter be tender and rigid, the assumption may be made that the condition is a local peritonitis, though a stethoscope applied to the lower part of the chest might possibly reveal the fact that the origin of the symptoms was a diaphragmatic pleurisy.

The exact order or method of examination which one may follow is a matter of individual choice or preference, but the routine followed by the writer is indicated and described in the succeeding chapters.

4. Many examinations of the abdomen are imperfect because the practitioner does not act upon the important *principle of applying his knowledge of anatomy*. It is well to cultivate the habit of thinking anatomically in every case where the knowledge of structural relations can be put to advantage. There are very few abdominal cases in which this cannot be done. Application of anatomy makes diagnosis more interesting and more rational. The explanation of some doubtful point, the differentia-

tion of the possible causes of a pain, the determination of the exact site of a diseased focus, often depend
upon small anatomical points. One is accustomed

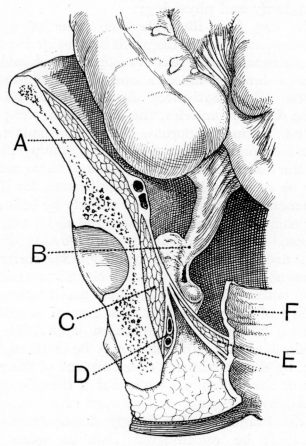

FIG. 2.—Drawing to show anatomical parts concerned in obturator
test. A = ilio-psoas; B = inflamed appendix with small abscess;
C = obturator internus; E = levator ani; D = Alcock's canal;
F = rectum.

to marvel at the accurate diagnoses of the neurolo-
gist, which are for the most part based upon a
sound knowledge of microscopic anatomy. Nothing

like the same accuracy is yet achieved in abdominal diagnosis, but it is the writer's faith that such will come in time by carefully applying the knowledge of anatomy and physiology.

One can best illustrate the value of applied anatomy in abdominal diagnosis by considering those structures which are least variable in their position —the voluntary muscles and the cerebro-spinal nerves. The frontispiece shows well the position of the different muscles, the diaphragm, the psoas, the quadratus lumborum, the erector spinæ, the lateral abdominal muscles, the recti, the pyriformis and the obturator internus. Each of these muscles may be of valuable clinical significance, for if any of them be irritated directly or reflexly by inflammatory changes it becomes tender and rigid, and pain is caused when the muscle fibres are moved. Everyone is acquainted with the rigidity of the rectus and lateral abdominal muscles when there is a subjacent inflammatory focus, but few take much note of the rigidity of the diaphragm in a case of subphrenic abscess, because the diaphragm is invisible and impalpable. Its immobility may be deduced, however, by the impairment of movement of the upper part of the abdominal wall, and if the X-rays are available the rigidity and absence of movement of the diaphragm can be directly demonstrated.

It will be remembered that in some cases of appendicitis and other conditions affecting the psoas muscle there is flexion of the thigh, due to contraction of the muscle consequent on direct or reflex irritation, but how often does anyone test the slighter degrees of such irritation by causing the patient to lie on the opposite side and extending

to the full the thigh on the affected side ?   Again, the
obturator internus is covered by a dense fascia and

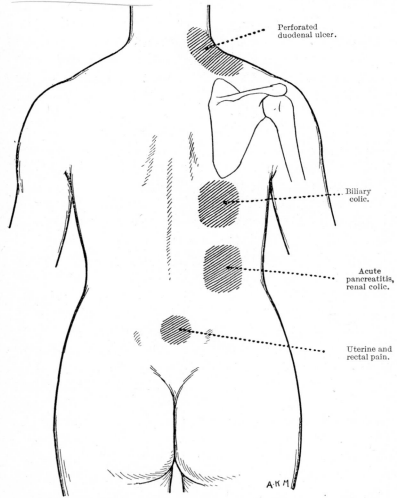

Perforated
duodenal ulcer.

Biliary
colic.

Acute
pancreatitis,
renal colic.

Uterine and
rectal pain.

A·K·M

FIG. 3.—Diagram to show the sites on posterior surface of body to which
pain is referred in acute abdominal conditions.

is not readily irritated by pelvic inflammation ; but
if there be an abscess (e.g. one caused by a ruptured

appendix) immediately adjacent to the fascia, pain will be caused if the muscle be put through its full movement by rotating the flexed thigh inward to its extreme limit.   The pain is referred to the hypogastrium.   This sign is not present in every case of pelvic appendicitis, and may occur in other pelvic conditions, such as pelvic hæmatocele, but when present it denotes a definite pathological change. (Fig. 2.)

The application of the knowledge of the anatomical course and distribution of the segmental nerves is also important.   When a patient complains of loin-pain radiating to the corresponding testis one remembers the embryological fact that the testis is developed in the same region as the kidney ; and though the former travels to the scrotum just before birth, yet in suffering it shows its sympathy with and serves as an indicator for the intra-abdominal structure which was developed near it.   Of course, pain referred to the testicle does not always denote primary genito-urinary disease.   It is probable that the main nerve-supply to the vermiform appendix comes from the tenth dorsal segment, so that pain in one or both testicles may be caused by such a condition as appendicitis.   The dorsal distribution of referred pain should also be noted. (See Fig. 3.)

Another segmental pain of great importance is that referred from the diaphragm.   The diaphragm begins to develop in the region of the fourth cervical segment from which is obtained the major part of its muscle-fibres.   Nerve-fibres, mainly from the fourth cervical nerve, accompany the muscle-fibres and constitute the phrenic nerve.   The growth of

the thoracic contents causes the muscle to be displaced caudal-wards, and it finally takes up its
position at the lower outlet of the thorax.   The

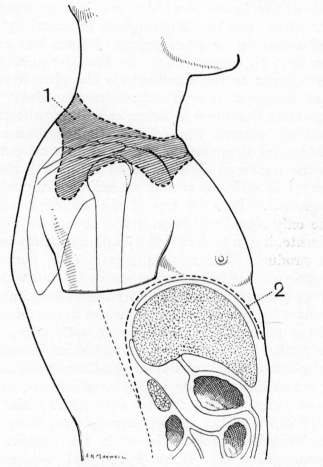

Fig. 4.—Diagram to indicate (1) the shoulder area in which phrenic
irritation may cause pain ; (2) line of diaphragm.

phrenic nerves elongate to accommodate themselves
to the displaced muscle. From the diagnostic
point of view the separation from the original

position is extremely valuable, for if in upper
abdominal or lower thoracic lesions pain be felt, or
hyperæsthesia be detected in the region of distribution of the fourth cervical nerve, it is a strong presumption that the diaphragm is irritated by some
inflammatory or other lesion. Hilton was one of
the first to suggest that the shoulder-pain might
be referred to the shoulder via the phrenic nerve,
and Ferguson proved experimentally sixty years
ago that the phrenic nerve contained afferent as
well as efferent fibres. Yet the significance in
abdominal diagnosis of constant or intermittent pain
in the region of distribution of the fourth cervical
nerves is still either not understood or seriously
neglected. Pain on top of the shoulder may be
the only signal which an inarticulate liver abscess,
threatening to perforate the diaphragm, may be able
to produce. The agonizing pain of a perforated
gastric ulcer is felt on top of one or both shoulders in
proportion as the acrid and irritating fluid impinges
against the diaphragm and irritates the terminations
of the phrenic nerves on one or both sides. Pain
may also be referred to the shoulder in cases of
subphrenic abscess, diaphragmatic pleurisy, acute
pancreatitis, gall-stones, ruptured spleen, and in
some cases of appendicitis with peritonitis. The
pain is felt either in the supraspinous fossa, over
the acromion or clavicle, or in the subclavicular
fossa. (Fig. 4.) There is clinical evidence to
support the opinion that there is a correspondence
of nerve-distribution over the diaphragm and over
the acromio-clavicular region, so that lesions affecting a certain portion of the diaphragm cause pain
over the corresponding part of the shoulder area on

the same side of the body. Pain on top of both shoulders indicates a median diaphragmatic irritation. The shoulder-pain is apt to be overlooked, since the patient may term it " rheumatism." (Fig. 5.)

Errors in diagnosis also result from want of

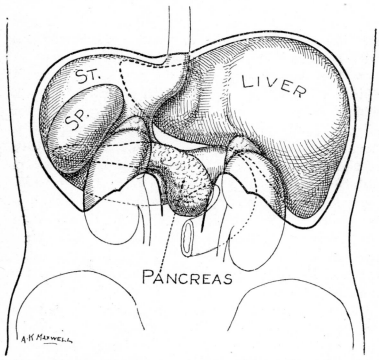

FIG. 5.—Diagram to show viscera in relation with diaphragm. (Posterior view with back part of diaphragm cut away.)   *St.* = stomach; *Sp.* = spleen.

appreciation of another anatomical point, i.e. the lack of representation in the muscular abdominal wall of the segments which form the pelvis, so that irritation of the pelvic nerves (e.g. from pelvic peritonitis) causes no abdominal-wall rigidity. Peritonitis commencing deep in the pelvis may therefore be unaccompanied by any rigidity of the hypogastric abdominal wall.

The above illustrations serve to demonstrate the importance of applying knowledge of anatomy in abdominal diagnosis. It is unnecessary to emphasize the great importance that a thorough acquaintance with the normal size, position, and relations of the abdominal viscera has in connexion with the elucidation of abdominal disease.

5. The localization of inflammatory lesions is aided **particularly** by knowledge of anatomy, whilst in obstructive lesions the application of physiological knowledge plays perhaps a more important part. The question of shock, the nature of the movements and sensations of the intestine, not to mention the various and important physiological tests demonstrating visceral functional derangements, are all intimately bound up with the problem of the acute abdomen. Very important also is the study of the effect of various toxins upon the viscera and the neuro-muscular reflexes of the abdomen.

A very large number of urgent abdominal cases are accompanied by pain due to abnormal conditions in tubes whose walls are composed mainly of unstriped muscle-fibres. There is no high-grade sensibility in such tubes. It is possible to crush, cut, or tear intestine without the fully conscious patient experiencing any pain, yet everyone is aware that pain does take origin from the intestine. What induces such pain ? The required stimulus is stretching or distension of the tube or excessive contraction against resistance. Evidence of pain arising from a tube of involuntary muscle is there-

fore indicative of local distension, either by gas
or fluid or of vigorous contraction.   In mild degrees
in the intestine this is commonly called flatulence,
in greater degrees in either intestinal, biliary, renal,
or uterine tubes it is called colic.   Severe colic
always indicates obstruction causing local distension or violent peristaltic contraction.   It occurs in
paroxysms, and the pain, which is often of an
excruciating nature, is referred to the sympathetic
centre from which the nerves come, and also to the
segmental distribution corresponding to the part
of the spinal cord from which the sympathetic
nerves to the affected viscus are derived.   Colic
of the small intestine causes pain referred chiefly
to the epigastric and umbilical regions, whilst large-
intestine colic is usually referred to the hypogastrium.   The pain of biliary colic is usually felt
more in the right subscapular region, whilst that
of renal colic is felt in the loin and sometimes radiates to the corresponding testicle.   Severe colic is
certainly one of the most terrible trials to which
a human being can be subjected.   The excessive
stimulation of the nerve-centres is often reflected
into motor channels so that the patients frequently
fling themselves about, twist and double themselves
up in a characteristic way.   If, therefore, a patient
gets paroxysms of pain which are accompanied
by the most violent restlessness of agony, the
chances are that the condition is some form of
obstruction and not peritonitis, for in the latter
condition movement generally increases the pain.

   The physiology of shock is still a subject of dis-
cussion, and rather widely differing opinions are
held thereon.   But whatever views be held as to

A.A.—2

the exact metabolic or nervous changes which are responsible for the symptoms, we believe that few would fail to allow that in acute abdominal disease two varieties can be recognized. One is the initial or primary shock due to sudden stimulation of many nerve-terminals, as in the perforation of a gastric ulcer into the general peritoneal cavity, or the severe stimulation of a few, as for example in severe biliary colic.

The second variety of shock, which might be termed late, toxic, or secondary shock, is that in which somewhat similar symptoms arise at a later stage, partly no doubt from severe afferent nerve stimulation, sometimes from loss of fluid from the blood-vessels into the extra-vascular tissues, but chiefly from the absorption of poisons which directly affect the higher nerve centres. The terminal stage of this secondary shock is commonly termed collapse.

Between primary and secondary shock, as here described, there is often an interval, a latent period, during which the observer may easily be deceived. In many cases of perforated ulcer the sudden stimulation of the nerve-endings in the peritoneum or subperitoneal tissue causes severe shock. After a time the nerve-equilibrium is restored and the pulse, respiration, temperature, and appearance of the patient improve so much that one might think the pathological process was stayed or improving. Soon, however, the symptoms of peritonitis dominate the scene, and one realizes that the calm period was but that of physiological reaction. This period is the cause of many mistakes in diagnosis.

Another physiological fact of importance is

that hyperæsthesia and tenderness due to irritation of nerves by a unilateral lesion are not usually felt on the opposite side of the body. For example, a right-sided pleurisy will sometimes cause tenderness and rigidity in the right, but not in the left iliac region. If the fingers pressed well into the left iliac fossa and pushed deeply towards the right side across the middle line evoke tenderness, it will indicate a deep inflammatory lesion in the right iliac region.

6. In diagnosing acute abdominal disease it is *always necessary to exclude medical diseases* before concluding that the condition is one needing surgical intervention. Certain aspects of disease which may simulate the acute abdomen can only be learnt either in the medical wards of a large hospital or in an extensive general medical practice. Typhoid fever, cardiac derangements, chronic interstitial nephritis and arterio-sclerosis, cirrhosis of the liver, tuberculous peritonitis—all these and many other medical diseases will sooner or later cause doubt in abdominal diagnosis. The one who would be prepared thoroughly to examine and correctly to diagnose the acute abdomen must at any rate know how to use, even if he be not expert in the use of, the ophthalmoscope, the sphygmomanometer, the leucocytometer, and the stethoscope—not to mention the urine-testing apparatus.

Opening of the abdomen is not to be advised with too light a heart. The dextrous hand must not be allowed to reach before the imperfect judgment. Abdominal section is only to be made on the recommendation of a mature judgment after a thorough examination. It is regrettable to have to say afterwards that one did not know that there was severe albuminuria, or that the patient was the subject of tabes dorsalis, or that the lungs were not examined. Perhaps the traditional precedence of the physician over the surgeon is not without its significance even to-day.

If, however, after careful examination one comes to the conclusion that there is within the abdomen the early stage of a pathological process which tends to get worse and which is amenable to surgical treatment, there should be no hesitation in recommending operation, even though the patient and his relatives may not think the condition serious. Correct diagnosis is the basis of firm counsel.

CHAPTER II

METHOD OF DIAGNOSIS : (I) THE HISTORY

In diagnosing acute abdominal disease it is well to have a routine method of examination, not to be slavishly followed, but to be modified according to circumstances. Increasing experience enables one to dispense with some parts of the examination—for example, a woman collapsed and blanched with obvious intra-abdominal hæmorrhage is not to be subjected to an examination which entails a risk of producing further hæmorrhage—but in general, and when urgency permits, routine method is desirable.

The accompanying scheme, to be filled in during the examination of the patient, was used by me at St. Mary's Hospital for some years, and may be found useful as a general guide. There are two main sections in this scheme : one devoted to the ascertaining of the history of the condition for which advice is sought ; the other reserved for the result of the physical examination of the patient. The former includes both the story of the present illness and any more remote disease which may possibly bear upon the present derangement.

History of present condition.—It can be confidently asserted that a large number of acute abdominal conditions could be diagnosed by considering carefully the history of onset. That is only possible, however, when each symptom is carefully

21

FORM FOR ACUTE ABDOMINAL CASES

Patient's Name ....*Sex*........ *Age* ...

Address ....

Date and time of examination ....

HISTORY OF PRESENT CONDITION

EXACT TIME OF ONSET.   MODE OF ONSET.—Acute or Gradual.

PAIN.—(*a*) Situation at first.   (*b*) Has it shifted ?
    (*c*) Character.   (*d*) Any radiation ?
    (*e*) Pain on micturition.

VOMITING.—Before—at same time—or some hours after pain.
    How often ?   Character of vomit

NAUSEA.

BOWELS.—Regular usually ?   When last open.
    Diarrhœa ?   Any blood in motions ?

MENSTRUATION.—Exact date of last period.
    Whether last period + or —.   Painful or not.

PAST HISTORY

Any serious previous illness ?

INDIGESTION.—If so, how long after meals before pain comes.
    Jaundice.   Melæna.   Hæmatemesis.
    Hæmaturia.   Loss of weight.

CONFINEMENTS (if any).

PRESENT CONDITION

PULSE.   BLOOD-PRESSURE.   RESP.   TEMP.

GENERAL APPEARANCE.

ABDOMEN.—Pain.   Tenderness.   Cutaneous.   Rigidity.   Distension.
                  Hyperæsthesia.
    Movement on respiration.   Tumour or external
    Free fluid.   hernia.
    Thigh-rotation test.   Liver dullness.

RECTAL EXAMINATION.

CHEST EXAMINATION.

SPINE.   KNEE-JERKS.   PUPILS.

URINE.—Blood.   Pus.   Albumin   Sugar.

VAGINAL DISCHARGE.

BIMANUAL EXAMINATION   X-RAY EXAMINATION.

appraised in relation to the other symptoms, so that its significance is properly understood. We shall therefore consider each item in the case-form separately.

Age.—To know a patient's age is helpful, since the incidence of certain conditions is limited within certain years. Acute intussusception in temperate climates occurs generally in infants under two years of age ; appendicitis seldom occurs in infancy, but is most common in young adolescents. Obstruction of the large intestine by a cancerous stricture is seldom seen before thirty, is infrequent before forty, but is the commonest cause of intestinal obstruction in persons over forty years of age. Acute pancreatitis is seldom or never seen in those under middle age. A perforated gastric ulcer is a great rarity in anyone under fifteen years. Conditions such as cholecystitis or a twisted pedicle of an ovarian cyst may occur in childhood, though much more common in adult life. All the acute conditions which are due to derangements of the developing ovum or its surroundings are naturally only found in women between the limits of the child-bearing period.

Exact time and mode of onset.—It is frequently possible for the patient to fix the exact time at which the pain started. The awakening out of sleep by acute abdominal pain is so startling that it is not forgotten. Acute appendicitis very commonly, and perforation of a gastric ulcer not infrequently, commence in this manner. It is no ordinary pain which begins thus.

Many acute conditions appear to be precipitated by some slight exertion or by the internal disturbance caused by the energetic working of an aperient. Many cases of incipient appendicitis become much worse soon after the administration of castor oil or its equivalent. The temporary increase of intra-abdominal tension caused by any slight straining effort may cause the giving way of the thin floor of a gastric ulcer, or the rupture of a pregnant Fallopian tube.

It is also important to determine whether the condition began immediately after some injury; apparently trivial abdominal injuries may be accompanied or followed by serious lesions.

The **acuteness of onset** gives some indication of the severity of the lesion. Ask if the patient fainted or fell down collapsed at the onset of symptoms. Perforation of a gastric or duodenal ulcer and acute pancreatitis are the only two abdominal conditions likely to cause a man to faint. In a woman the rupture of an ectopic gestation usually causes fainting.

Many cases of intestinal obstruction are gradual in onset, culminating in an acute crisis. Strangulation of the gut, however, is accompanied by very acute symptoms from the first. The symptoms due to torsion of the pedicle of an ovarian cyst are also usually acute from the start.

To know the exact time of onset is useful in estimating the probable pathological changes that have ensued; for example, it is not usual for an appendix to perforate within twenty-four hours of the onset of symptoms, so, unless the symptoms definitely point to diffuse peritonitis, one may give a better prognosis for the operation of appendicectomy if performed within that time. Again, it is only by ascertaining the precise moment of onset that one can tell whether the apparent well-being of the patient corresponds to the stage of reaction which is seen in some conditions—notably in patients with perforated gastric or duodenal ulcer.

Pain.—The greatest importance attaches to the very careful consideration of the onset, distribution, and character of the pain.

Situation of the pain at first.—When the peritoneal cavity is flooded suddenly by either blood (from a ruptured tubal gestation-sac), or pus (e.g. from a ruptured pyosalpinx), or acrid fluid (from a perforated gastric ulcer), the pain is frequently said to be felt " all over the abdomen " from the first. But the maximum intensity of pain at the onset is likely to be in the upper abdomen in the last-mentioned and in the lower abdomen in the two former conditions. In perforated duodenal ulcer the pain may be at first more acute in the right hypochondrium and right lumbar and iliac regions, owing to the irritating fluid passing down chiefly on the right side of the abdomen.

Pain arising from the small intestine, whether due to simple colic, organic obstruction or strangulation, is always felt first and chiefly in the epigastric and umbilical areas of the abdomen, i.e. in the zone of distribution of the ninth to eleventh thoracic nerves which supply small intestine via the common mesentery. Remembering that the appendicular nerves are derived from the same source as those which supply the small intestine, it is not surprising that the pain at the onset of an attack of appendicitis is usually felt in the epigastrium. When small intestine is adherent to the abdominal wall, pain caused by its peristaltic movement is referred to that part of the abdominal wall to which the gut is adherent.

The pain of large-gut affections is more commonly felt at first in the hypogastrium, or, in the case of the cæcum and ascending and descending colon, when the meso-cæcum or meso-colon is very short or wanting, at the actual site of the lesion.

The shifting or localization of the pain is often significant. After a blow on the upper part of the abdomen, if local pain at the site of injury be the first complaint, but in a few hours the pain be referred more to the hypogastrium, one must suspect rupture of intestine and consequent gravitation of the escaping fluid to the pelvis. Similarly, localization of pain in the right iliac fossa some hours after acute epigastric pain is usually due to appendicitis—though occasionally the same sequence is seen with a perforated pyloric or duodenal ulcer, or in a case of acute pancreatitis.

The character of the pain is occasionally a help as to the nature or seriousness of the condition. The general burning pain of a perforated gastric ulcer, the agony of an acute pancreatitis, the sharp constricting pain which takes away the breath in an attack of biliary colic, and the griping pain in many cases of intestinal obstruction contrast with the acute aching of many cases of appendicitis with abscess, or the constant dull fixed pain of a pyonephrosis.

Radiation of the pain is frequently diagnostic. This is specially true of the colics in which pain radiates to the area of distribution of the nerves coming from that segment of the spinal cord which supplies the affected part. Thus in biliary colic the pain is frequently referred to the region just under the inferior angle of the right scapula (eighth dorsal segment), whilst renal colic is frequently felt in the testicle of the same side.

In many conditions of the upper abdomen and lower thorax pain is referred to the top of the shoulder on the same side as the lesion (see Chapter I), and special inquiry should always be made as to pain or tenderness over the supra-spinous fossa, the acromion, or the clavicle.

It is always well to *ascertain if the pain is influenced by respiration.* Pleuritic pain is usually worse on taking a deep inspiration, and is diminished or stopped during a respiratory pause. Biliary colic may cause inhibition of movement of the diaphragm, and the pain may be increased by a forced respiration. In many cases of peritonitis, intra-peritoneal abscess, or abdominal distension due to intestinal obstruction, pain will be caused on inspiration.

Special varieties of pain.—It is necessary to ask if there be any pain during the act of micturition, for the presence or absence of such pain is frequently of great significance. In addition to its causation by primarily urinary conditions, e.g. pyelitis, stone in the kidney or ureter, or acute hydronephrosis, pain on micturition is not infrequently caused by a pelvic abscess which lies close to the bladder, or by an inflamed appendix which irritates the right ureter. Pain in the corresponding testicle may accompany renal colic, but testicular pain may occasionally occur with appendicitis.

Vomiting.—In acute abdominal lesions, apart from acute gastritis, vomiting is almost always due to one or more of three causes :

(1) *Severe irritation of the nerves of the peritoneum or mesentery,* e.g. consequent on the

perforation of a gastric ulcer or of a gangrenous appendix, or torsion of an ovarian cyst pedicle.

(2) *Obstruction of an involuntary muscular tube*, whether it be the biliary duct, the ureter, the uterine canal, or the intestine.

(3) The action of absorbed toxins upon the medullary centres.

(1) It needs little imagination to picture the intensity of stimulation of the nerve-endings in the peritoneum by the acid gastric juice flowing freely into the peritoneal cavity, nor is it surprising that a patient should vomit very soon after the onset of such irritation.   But the rapid and copious pouring out of diluting fluid from the irritated peritoneal surface soon dilutes the acid gastric juice and lessens the irritation, so that vomiting is seldom persistent after the perforation of a gastric ulcer.

In acute pancreatitis the cœliac plexus is so intimately associated with the inflamed organ that the reflex stimulus is very great and vomiting is therefore very severe.   It is frequently persistent, since there is no mitigation of the severe stimulus apart from operation or gangrene of the organ.

Strangulation of a coil of intestine and torsion of the pedicle of an ovarian cyst are examples of sudden catastrophes in which sudden and severe stimulation of many sympathetic nerves causes vomiting to occur early and to be persistent.

(2) Stretching of involuntary muscles causes pain, and if the stretching be extreme, vomiting occurs.   Obstruction of any of the muscular tubes causes peristaltic contraction and consequent

stretching of the muscle-wall due to distension, and vomiting is therefore common with such obstruction. This is well seen in all the colics, biliary, renal, intestinal, and uterine. Behind the obstruction the tube becomes somewhat dilated, and, as each peristaltic wave passes along, the tension and stretching of the muscular fibres are temporarily increased, so that the pain of colic comes usually in spasms. Vomiting usually occurs at the height of the pain.

In intestinal obstruction there is the additional factor that the contents of the intestine are mechanically prevented from progressing onward, and a reversed current may be set up, possibly as the result of antiperistalsis. The contents of the intestine, sometimes as far down as the site of obstruction, are therefore vomited.

(3) Toxic vomiting is seen in cases of septic peritonitis. It is possible that in intestinal obstruction the vomiting is partially due to the effect of absorbed poisons upon the medullary centres.

The relationship of pain to vomiting.—It is important always to inquire the exact time of vomiting relative to the onset of pain. In sudden and severe stimulation of the peritoneum or mesentery vomiting is early, coming on soon after the pain. In acute obstruction of the ureter by a stone or of the bile-duct by a calculus vomiting is early, sudden, and violent. In intestinal obstruction the length of interval before vomiting ensues gives some indication as to how high in the gut the obstruction is situated. If the duodenum has become obstructed by a gall-stone, vomiting comes on almost as soon as the pain, and is for a time, and until the stone passes on, frequent and violent. If the lower end of the ileum be constricted (apart from strangulation, which leads to early vomiting), the vomiting may not occur for four or more hours, according to the acuteness of the stoppage. In large-bowel obstruction the vomiting is usually quite a late feature and sometimes may not occur at all, though nausea is often present at a much earlier stage.

In appendicitis pain almost always precedes the vomiting, usually by three or four hours, sometimes by twelve or twenty-four hours or even longer. Rarely indeed does the vomiting occur simultaneously with the onset of pain, and very rarely does the pain start after the vomiting.

The frequency of the vomiting usually varies directly as the acuteness of the condition. Frequent vomiting *at the onset* of an attack of acute appendicitis usually means that the appendix is distended on the distal side of a stricture or concretion, and signals the immediate danger of perforation. Frequent vomiting later in the course of an appendicitis usually means extension of peritonitis.

There are, however, many serious abdominal conditions in which vomiting is either infrequent, slight, or absent. Internal hæmorrhage from a ruptured ectopic gestation is often accompanied by little or no vomiting. After the initial shock due to perforation of a gastric or duodenal ulcer there is often a latent period before symptoms of peritonitis assert themselves. During this period vomiting may not occur and nausea may not be complained of.

In obstruction of the large intestine vomiting is

a late or infrequent symptom. This is very noticeable in cases of intussusception, where the absence
of vomiting may deceive as to the acuteness and
danger of the condition. When vomiting occurs in
undoubted obstruction of the large intestine it is
generally due to the failure of the ileo-caecal valve
allowing the back-pressure to distend the lower
ileum.

In obstruction high up in the small intestine
vomiting is frequent and copious in quantity.

The character of the vomit needs to be noted.
In acute gastritis, which in severe cases may give
rise to alarming abdominal symptoms, the vomit
consists of the contents of the stomach possibly
mixed with a little bile. In the colics the vomit is
commonly bilious. In cases of severe sympathetic
shock, such as occurs with acute torsion of a viscus,
it is common for the patient to retch frequently
but vomit very little.

In intestinal obstruction the character of the
vomited material varies. First the gastric contents, then bilious material, then greenish yellow,
yellow, and finally brown fæculent smelling fluid is
ejected. Fæculent vomit is pathognomonic of
obstruction of the intestine—either mechanical or
paralytic.

Nausea and *loss of appetite* are induced in many
people who do not vomit. In some patients it
appears to need a greater stimulus to produce
vomiting than in others. In the same person
different grades of the same kind of stimulus may
produce anorexia, nausea, or vomiting. Therefore
it is always important to inquire for the two former
as well as the latter. *Acute* loss of appetite is

always significant. In a child especially a sudden
distaste for food accompanied by abdominal pain
should always cause one to make a very careful
examination for appendicitis. In questioning a
child it is well to find out the last meal that the
child really enjoyed, and the first for which it had
no eagerness.

Bowels.—It is, of course, important to investigate
the condition of the bowels, but it is unwise to
attach too much importance to the simple fact of
constipation, unless accompanied by other symptoms. What is of greater importance is any significant departure from previously normal action of
the bowel. In a person who is accustomed to a
regular action of the bowels every day, the occurrence of constipation for several days may be of
serious import, especially if accompanied by
abdominal pain or flatulence.

The passage of several small loose motions
amounting almost to diarrhœa is common at the
onset of many cases of appendicitis in children.
*When hypogastric pain and diarrhœa are followed
by hypogastric tenderness and constipation suspect
a pelvic abscess.* Tenesmus is sometimes a complaint in cases of pelvic abscess.

The presence of obvious blood or slime in the
motions is to be asked after and looked for. The
significance of blood and mucus in the rectum in the
diagnosis of intussusception is well known.

Menstruation.—Since pregnancy and the derangements thereof play so large a part in the health
and disease of women, it is essential to inquire into
the regularity of menstruation. It is not sufficient to ask whether the periods are regular, the

exact date of the last period must be ascertained and any irregularity noted. Antedating or post-dating of the normal period by a few days, or a longer or more profuse loss or the reverse, must be noted. Many patients with tubal gestation take the uterine loss which occurs at the time of threatening tubal abortion or rupture as the normal menstrual loss, if the hæmorrhage happens to coincide with the time of the usual monthly period. In such cases, however, it is nearly always possible by careful questioning to ascertain that the loss is in some way abnormal.

Pain accompanying the period of a woman who is not usually subject to dysmenorrhœa should make one think of threatening early abortion, tubal gestation, or some condition unassociated with pregnancy.

Past history.—It is well to inquire concerning any previous illness, e.g. typhoid fever, peritonitis, appendicitis, or pneumonia, which may possibly have a bearing on the present illness.

Since many if not most abdominal pains are loosely termed indigestion, inquiry should be directed as to the occurrence of any pain which has any relationship to the taking of food. Pain which comes on two or two and a half hours after food would suggest duodenal ulcer. Constant epigastric pain made worse by the taking of food would make one suspicious of carcinoma or chronic ulcer of the stomach. Epigastric or right hypochondriac pain irregularly related to meals is in keeping with the presence of gall-stones.

Previous attacks of jaundice, melæna, hæmatemesis, and hæmaturia must briefly be inquired after, and it is well to find out if any great and known loss of weight has occurred.

Previous residence in tropical climes and any dysenteric history should be ascertained.

In a woman previous confinements or pregnancies should be noted.

CHAPTER III

METHOD OF DIAGNOSIS : (II) THE EXAMINA-
TION OF THE PATIENT

The general appearance.—The facial expression of
the patient will on occasion furnish valuable evidence of the serious nature of the pain of which he
complains. The pale or livid face with sweating
brow of a patient suffering from the initial shock of
a perforated gastric ulcer, acute pancreatitis, or
acute strangulation of gut is sufficiently distinctive,
whilst the deathly pallor and gasping respiration of
a woman with internal hæmorrhage from rupture
of a tubal gestation leave little doubt as to the
diagnosis. But appearances are often deceptive,
and in connexion with acute abdominal disease it is
important ever to keep in mind the reaction from
initial shock which commonly occurs and renders
latent even the most serious internal conditions.
Most surgeons of experience have seen patients
suffering from perforation of a gastric ulcer who
gave no indication from complexion or facial expression of the serious intra-abdominal condition
from which they were suffering. The so-called
abdominal facies is not infrequently absent in an
abdominal case. In the majority of cases of early
appendicitis the facial appearance of the patient
does not help at all. But in the late stages of all
varieties of acute abdominal disease the face tells
the observer much that he ought to know, but is

sorry to learn. The dull gaze of the eyes and the ashen countenance of one suffering from severe toxæmia, or the sunken cheeks and hollow-eyed aspect of the patient who has been vomiting repeatedly from internal obstruction or advanced peritonitis can always be recognized by the skilled clinician.

The back of the observer's hand placed on the patient's nose and cheek will often determine whether shock is present or collapse impending, for a cold nose and cheek, due to failing capillary circulation, are usually indicative of one or the other.

If the alæ nasi are observed to be moving the attention should always be particularly directed to the thorax, for a high temperature with moving alæ nasi generally means pneumonia. It must be remembered, however, that any abdominal condition which in any way impedes the movement of the diaphragm may be accompanied by movement of the alæ.

The attitude in bed is noteworthy. The restlessness of those suffering from severe colic or from intra-peritoneal hæmorrhage contrasts with the immobility and dislike of movement evinced by the majority of those suffering from peritonitis. Ask a patient suffering from a perforated gastric ulcer to turn on to his side, and one sees at once the difficulty, circumspection, and pain with which the movement is accomplished. With extensive peritonitis the knees are frequently drawn up to relax the abdominal tension, whilst any inflammatory condition in contact with the psoas muscle causes a flexion of the corresponding thigh.

In the early stages of many pathological states of the abdomen, however, no great help is obtainable from observing the attitude.

The pulse is too optimistic a friend to be relied upon for guidance, either in diagnosis or prognosis, in the early stages of acute abdominal disease. Exception must be made of the weak rapid pulse of the initial shock-stage of many of the abdominal catastrophes, but one can prove the unreliability of the pulse as a general guide by stating what every operator of experience knows, i.e. that the pulse *may* be regular in force and normal in frequency, even though there be an acutely inflamed appendix, or a ruptured intestine, or an obstructed coil of gut, or even (rarely) an acutely inflamed pancreas causing the abdominal pain. A normal pulse does not necessarily indicate a normal condition of the abdomen.

On the other hand, an increase in frequency of the pulse is a constant accompaniment of the more advanced stages of peritonitis and hæmorrhage, and after abdominal injury the careful observance of the pulse hour by hour is of great value in estimating the nature or seriousness of the intra-abdominal trouble. In advancing peritonitis, also, there is frequently a slight irregularity in force and an occasional intermittence of the pulse which may be significant.

The pulse of late peritonitis—small, hard, rapid so as to be almost uncountable—is usually a terminal event, and is always of bad prognostic significance.

If acute abdominal disease is to be diagnosed in the early stages, it must first be realized by the practitioner, who will see the case at the beginning, that many, if not most, patients with serious acute lesions of the abdomen have a normal pulse for a considerable time during the early stage.

The respiration-rate is chiefly of importance in differentiating between an abdominal and a thoracic condition. If the respiration-rate be raised to double the normal at the inception of the illness, the causative lesion is probably thoracic in origin. In general peritonitis, however, or in cases of intestinal obstruction with great distension, or in severe intra-abdominal hæmorrhage, the breathing may be much more hurried than usual, and with some persons nervousness produces shallow and more rapid respiration. The pulse-respiration ratio is of greater value in diagnosis.

Temperature.—A sub-normal, normal, or raised temperature may accompany acute abdominal disease. All three may be recorded in the same case at different times. In any severe abdominal shock or in severe toxæmia the thermometer frequently registers as low as 95° F. or 96° F. This is the temperature, for example, often recorded at the onset of an attack caused by acute pancreatitis, acute intestinal strangulation, perforated gastric ulcer, or severe intra-peritoneal hæmorrhage.

At the onset of an attack of acute appendicitis the temperature is usually normal, but within a few hours it generally rises steadily to about 100° F. or 101° F. When perforation occurs the temperature usually goes a little higher, but sometimes the absorption of depressing toxins may bring down the temperature to normal, or even sub-normal.

A normal temperature is often seen in the re-action stage of a perforated gastric ulcer.

The reaction stage of a ruptured ectopic gestation is usually accompanied by irregular but not high fever.

In intestinal obstruction the temperature is, as a rule, normal or sub-normal. If any patient with abdominal pain is found to have a temperature of 104° or 105° at the onset of the illness, the thorax or the kidney is very likely the seat of the disease. High fever is quite unusual during the early stages of acute abdominal disease.

Tongue.—Though usual it is by no means invari-able to find the tongue furred in acute abdominal conditions. In acute appendicitis and acute in-testinal obstruction there is usually a slight coat on the tongue and the breath is frequently foul.

The appearance of the tongue is a valuable guide in cases of uræmia, which may simulate intestinal obstruction. In renal failure the tongue is very dry, and heavily covered with a brownish fur, whilst there is a tendency for sordes to collect on the teeth.

ABDOMINAL EXAMINATION

Before examining the abdomen it is well to learn from the patient the exact place where the pain started, and if there has been any alteration in its location. The exact point of maximal pain should also be pointed out at the time of examination.

Inspection of the abdomen will reveal at a glance any abnormal local or general distension, and will in some cases determine the presence of a tumour or abdominal swelling. *All the hernial orifices must be inspected as a routine, and special attention directed to the femoral canal, where, in a fat subject, a small hernia is not difficult to overlook.*

The respiratory-movement of the abdominal wall is carefully to be noted, for any limitation indicates some rigidity of the diaphragm or abdominal muscles, or possibly undue distension. In the case of a perforated ulcer which has ruptured into the general peritoneal cavity, the abdominal wall hardly moves in any part on respiration, whilst in appendicitis the hypogastric zone, especially the right iliac area, will very frequently be seen immobile. In acute pancreatitis the epigastric zone may be motionless, and sometimes also the lower part of the abdominal wall. With biliary colic there is sometimes inhibition of the diaphragm so that the respiratory movement of the epigastric area of the abdominal wall is diminished.

In performing palpation of the abdomen it is hardly necessary to remind the reader that the hands should be warm, that the examination should be commenced by the hand at that part of the abdomen farthest removed from the point of maximum tenderness, and that gentle pressure should be made by the soft pulp of the fingers. Palpation determines the extent and intensity of the muscular defence or rigidity, locates any tender areas or hyperæsthetic patches, and determines the presence of any swelling. It is well to have the patient's thighs flexed while palpating the abdomen.

Muscular rigidity is a relative term. The contraction of the muscles may be firm, continuous, and "like a board," as in many cases of general peritonitis due to perforated ulcer, or the muscular fibres may not contract to any detectable extent till the fingers are gently pressed on the abdominal wall, when the muscles spring to attention to defend the subjacent inflamed parts. There is also an important mental factor in the production of abdominal-wall rigidity. In some sensitive children, and in some very apprehensive adolescents and adults, the abdominal wall is held very rigid even though there be very slight intra-abdominal cause for it.

In pelvic inflammatory lesions rigidity is often absent. In intestinal obstruction the muscles are not usually held rigid. In rigidity due to thoracic disease, if the muscle contraction be overcome by continuous pressure the abdominal pain is not usually increased, but if there be a subjacent inflamed area in the abdomen the pain becomes greater as the hand presses in and overcomes the muscular resistance.

It is exceedingly important to remember that muscular rigidity and resistance may be very slight even in the presence of serious peritonitis: (1) when the abdominal wall is very fat and flabby, and the muscles thin and weak; (2) when the patient is suffering from severe toxæmia, and the reflexes are dulled and diminished as the result of the absorbed toxins. It is noteworthy that the recti are usually more definitely rigid than the lateral abdominal muscles.

Hyperæsthesia.—Hyperæsthesia may be tested by pin-stroke or by light pinch. For routine use the testing by lightly stroking with the point of a pin is the best method to adopt. Care is taken to hold the pin at an acute angle to the skin so that it does not scratch. The abdominal skin is then stroked from above downwards in several vertical lines, first on the right side, then on the left. The patient is told to say at once if the pin-stroke feels sharper at any place. It is wise also to test the loin and posterior lumbar region in the same way. Hyperæsthesia may be detected (a) in the segmental distribution of that part of the spinal cord from which the affected viscus is innervated; (b) along the distribution of those peripheral nerves some of whose terminals are irritated by the inflammatory process. It will be found that cutaneous hyperæsthesia is present in half the number of acute abdominal conditions which present themselves for diagnosis. Hyperæsthesia nearly always indicates visceral or parietal peritoneal inflammation. It is not common to obtain hyperæsthesia in the upper abdomen. Most commonly the hypersensitive area lies below the umbilicus and varies from an iliac triangle on one or both sides to a small patch somewhere within the limits of the triangle. Occasionally a complete band stretches right back to the spine.

Though appendicitis is by far the most common abdominal disease which gives rise to hyperæsthesia in the lower part of the abdominal wall, yet cholecystitis, perforated duodenal ulcer, pyelitis, and various kinds of peritonitis may also cause cutaneous hypersensitiveness in the area above Poupart's ligament. It is, however, comparatively rare to find an iliac triangle of hyperæsthesia in any condition other than appendicitis. Hyperæsthesia is helpful when detected, but it is by no means a constant accompaniment of early disease, whilst in severely toxic cases it may also be absent.

Unimanual and bimanual palpation of the loins.—
This is of help in detecting renal or other loin-
swellings.

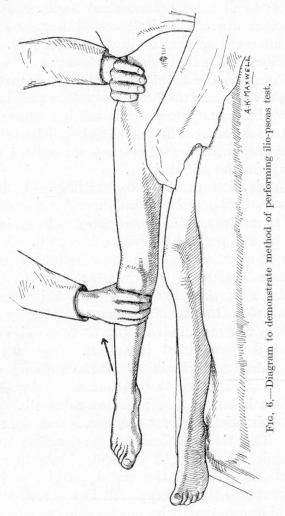

FIG. 6.—Diagram to demonstrate method of performing ilio-psoas test.

A.K.MAXWELL

The finger-tips of one or other hand are pressed
forward under the ribs of the corresponding side of

the patient's body. Resistance and tenderness without swelling indicate rigidity and sensitiveness of the quadratus lumborum and adjacent muscles, due probably to a tender inflammatory focus near-by. A perinephric abscess, an inflamed kidney, or a retro-cæcal inflamed appendix may give this sign.

In bimanual palpation the observer brings the other hand to the front of the loin, and can thus feel between the two hands any loin-swelling. A pyo- or hydro-nephrosis or a lumbar abscess can thus be detected. The patient should be asked to take a deep breath so that any movement of the swelling can be ascertained.

Determination of ilio-psoas rigidity.—It is well known that if there be an inflamed focus in relation to the psoas muscle the corresponding thigh is often flexed by the patient to relieve the pain. A lesser degree of such contraction (and irritation) can be determined often by putting the patient on the opposite side and extending the thigh on the affected side to the full extent. Pain will be caused by the manœuvre if the psoas be rigid from either reflex or direct irritation. (Fig. 6.) The value of the test is diminished if the abdominal wall be rigid. The psoas-test is not so easily elicited when the inflammation becomes subacute.

The estimation of liver-dullness is occasionally of value. The dullness due to the liver is usually obtainable in the right vertical nipple line from the fifth rib to below the costal margin, and from the seventh to the eleventh rib in the mid-axillary line. If in a patient who has no signs or symptoms of an atrophic liver, and in whom there is no abdominal distension, a resonant note be obtained on percussing in the normally dull area in front, or if in any case a resonant note be obtained in the normally dull liver-area in the axillary line, then there must be free gas in the peritoneal cavity due to the rupture of stomach or intestine. (The rare condition of pyo-pneumo-subphrenic abscess is usually a late result of a ruptured stomach.)

The determination of liver-dullness anteriorly is of no value in cases of great distension, for intestine may be pushed up and cause resonance higher than normal.

The determination of the existence of free fluid in the abdominal cavity by the proving of movable dullness is not of such great importance in diagnosing acute abdominal disease. There are very few acute abdominal conditions in which there is not some free fluid, and in those cases where there is an easily estimable amount of fluid there are usually other signs and symptoms which suffice. In the writer's experience it has seldom been necessary, and often inadvisable, to attempt to determine it. Free fluid in the abdomen may be serum, sero-pus, pus, or blood. If there be enough blood in the peritoneal cavity to cause movable dullness, it is unwise to move the patient about, and hæmorrhage should be evident from other symptoms. In peritonitis, with pouring out of a great deal of fluid, it causes pain to move the patient, and the test is usually unnecessary.

In intestinal obstruction the determination of free fluid is of some value and causes the patient little inconvenience. One flank is percussed while the patient lies on the back, and again after he has been turned over on to the opposite side. If the note changes from dull to resonant on changing position free fluid is present. The test is sometimes vitiated by the accumulation of fluid within the coils of obstructed intestine. Such fluid is often great in amount and, owing to the atony and dilatation of the gut, moves easily from one part of the abdomen to another with a changed position of the patient.

Examination of the pelvic cavity.—As important as the examination of the main abdominal cavity is the investigation of the pelvis. The following methods should be employed in addition to the previous examination.

Supra-pelvic palpation and percussion.—This will have been done generally in the usual abdominal palpation, but it is well to pay special attention to the supra-pelvic region. By pressing deeply behind one or other Poupart's ligament, or behind the pubis, one may detect either deep tenderness or a lump or a certain muscular resistance significant of deeper disease. A full bladder or enlarged uterus, a high pelvic abscess or an ovarian cyst, may be thus discovered.

Rectal digital examination is extremely important and informative. The patient may lie on the side or the back. (In peritonitis or hæmorrhage it is often unwise to alter the position from dorsal to lateral.) A rubber glove or finger-stall should be worn. The well-lubricated finger is gently introduced three or four inches up the rectal canal. By pressing forwards, backwards, upwards, and laterally, the whole lower pelvis can be explored.

Forwards in the male one can detect an enlarged prostate, a distended bladder, or diseased enlargement of the seminal vesicles. In the female one can palpate painful and painless swellings of Douglas' pouch, enlargements and displacements of the uterus.

By passing the finger well up the canal, stricture of the rectum due to cancer or fibrosis, or ballooning

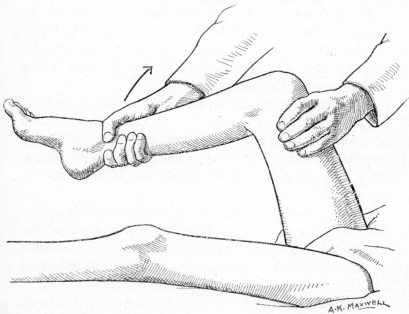

Fig. 7.—Diagram to illustrate method of performing obturator test.

of the canal below an obstruction can be ascertained. The apex of an intussusception may sometimes be felt.

It is important to test for tenderness on pressure against the pelvic peritoneum. (See Fig. 15, p. 102.)

Bulging of a pelvic abscess against the anterior rectal wall can readily be detected.

Laterally.—Tenderness due to an inflamed swollen

appendix or a small abscess on the lateral wall of the pelvis can be elicited.

Posteriorly.—Palpation will determine any tumour or inflammatory mass on the pyriformis, or in the hollow of the sacrum.

When the finger is withdrawn the presence on it of blood, slime, or pus should be noted.

In estimating the amount of pain caused by pressure upward on the pelvic peritoneum one must not be misled by the patient's expression of general discomfort, but must ascertain that the pain is due to pressure of the finger-tip.

Bimanual recto-abdominal or vagino-abdominal examination will determine the presence and position of any pelvic tumour or swelling. It is specially important to note the size and position of the uterus. Any fullness in Douglas' pouch should be carefully palpated.

In infants a bimanual recto-abdominal examination enables one to explore the lower part of the abdominal cavity thoroughly, and it may be possible to manipulate an intussusception between the fingers of the two hands.

Thigh-rotation test.[1]—When there is any inflamed mass adherent to the fascia over the obturator internus muscle, rotation of the flexed thigh, so as to put the irritated muscle through its full movements (especially internal rotation), will cause hypogastric pain. This sign should be tried especially when rectal examination is difficult, or for any reason inadvisable. (Fig. 7.) The sign is positive when a perforated appendix, a local abscess, and

---

[1] *Vide* Z. Cope, " The Obturator Test," *British Journal of Surgery,* vol. vii, 1920.

occasionally when a hæmatocele is in contact with the obturator internus, or when there is an accumulation of inflammatory fluid in the pelvis.

The chest should be thoroughly examined by the usual methods of inspection, palpation, percussion, and especially auscultation. By this means diaphragmatic pleurisy, early pneumonia, and pleural effusion will be detected.   The cardiac dullness must also be determined and the cardiac sounds auscultated.

Spine.—Any rigidity of or pain over the spinal column should be carefully observed, especially in children, in whom abdominal pain is frequently complained of during the course of spinal caries.

Knee-jerks and pupils.—In an adult no examination of a patient suffering acute abdominal pain is complete without a testing of the knee-jerks and the pupil-reactions.   If the pupils or even one pupil do not react to light, or if one or both knee-jerks are absent, search must be made for other signs of *tabes* so as to determine whether the pain is due to a visceral crisis.   Remember, however, that acute abdominal disease may exist in a tabetic subject.

Urine.—The importance of examination of the urine is well known, and constantly taught, but though the precept be acknowledged the practice is often at fault.   The presence of blood, pus, albumin, sugar, and bacteria should be ascertained. Not only is great light often thus thrown upon the diagnosis, but the finding of one or the other may qualify prognosis and alter treatment. Before operating on, and as a help in the diagnosis of, acute abdominal disease, it is sometimes wise to pass a catheter to ensure that the bladder is empty.

Blood-pressure.—The estimation of the blood-pressure is often of assistance in diagnosis of acute abdominal crises. It is chiefly in cases of internal hæmorrhage, shock, and circulatory failure following intestinal obstruction that a knowledge of the exact state of the blood-pressure is valuable. Both the systolic and the diastolic pressures need to be taken, for the most important figure to be known is the difference between the two, i.e. the pulse-pressure, which indicates the reserve power in the circulation. A low pulse-pressure is only found in the most serious states of collapse.

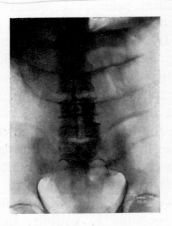

Fig. 8.—Radiogram showing dilatation of small intestine due to obstruction at the ileo-cæcal junction. The picture well demonstrates the ladder pattern.

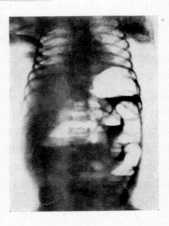

Fig. 9.—Radiogram of chest and abdomen of an infant four days old in whom congenital obstruction of the upper jejunum was correctly diagnosed by Dr. Gage on account of the gaseous distension of the stomach and the fluid levels in the jejunum.

X-ray examination.—With the increase in facilities for X-ray examination there is usually little difficulty in obtaining a radiograph of the abdomen

in cases which may require it.   Much information
may be obtained in cases of intestinal obstruction.
Local distension of coils of intestine in an otherwise undistended abdomen may point to small-bowel
obstruction, fluid levels may definitely demonstrate
a stoppage in the small intestine, and frequently
the outline of a distended colon will show the surgeon the exact site of the obstruction.   Most important of all in a case of suspected intussusception
a radiograph taken after the administration of a
barium enema will make the diagnosis certain.
(Figs. 8, 9 and 27.)

Auscultation of the abdomen is occasionally of
use in determining whether the normal sounds due
to intestinal movements are to be heard.   If no
sounds due to movement are heard it follows that
the intestines are in a state of paralysis due to ileus
or peritonitis.   Sometimes the nature of the sounds
may help one to conclude that gas is being forced
through an obstructed bowel.   Occasionally friction-
sounds consequent on peritonitis may be heard.
It is relevant here to remark that auscultation of the
abdomen was found by Blackburn and Rob to be of
the greatest assistance in determining whether or
not a gun-shot wound of the abdomen had caused
injury to the intestine ; they found that in the
presence of sounds due to intestinal movement it
was very rare to find any injury to the intestine.
They point out that the auscultation may have to
be repeated several times at intervals before making
up one's mind that movements are absent.   (*British
Journal of Surgery*, 1945, vol. 33, p. 46.)

Measurement of the abdomen has been used by
some surgeons to give information as to the progress

of a pathological lesion particularly as to increase of distension. The tape must of course be placed round the abdomen at the same level each time for the comparison to be of value. The author has not made use of this help, but agrees that it may be of assistance especially when X-rays may not be available.

CHAPTER IV

APPENDICITIS

General considerations.—If the mortality from appendicitis is to be reduced almost to vanishing-point, it is essential that the earliest signs and symptoms of the condition should be appreciated clearly; the view is accepted by most surgeons of experience that every case of acute appendicitis should be operated on within the first twenty-four hours from the onset, or as soon after as is possible. There are two reasons why cases are operated on later than this—either the patient may think that the symptoms are not serious enough to need medical advice, or the medical adviser may think the symptoms not typical of appendicitis or not serious enough to demand operation. It is clear that we have no remedy against the first cause save the education of the public, but in regard to the second something can be done by way of explaining that the so-called typical symptoms of appendicitis as given in the textbooks often indicate a somewhat advanced stage of the condition, and that it is impossible to say at the beginning of an attack whether it is likely to be mild or severe in type.

It is desirable and in most cases possible to diagnose appendicitis before peritonitis has set in, or at least before there is any more than that slight amount of congestion of the peritoneum which is commonly associated with any inflammatory process within the gut.

Pathological condition in relation to symptoms.— The different grades of inflammation of the vermiform appendix have for many years been well described and understood, though there is still in many quarters a lack of appreciation of the advanced pathological condition often coexistent with the initial symptoms, or at any rate with the initial complaint. Catarrh of the mucous membrane, parenchymatous inflammation of the whole wall, gangrene of the interior lining or of all but the peritoneal coat, any of these may coexist with symptoms so slight (but *not* indefinite) that they may be overlooked by the patient and thought of slight significance by the hurried and unobservant onlooker. Even rupture of the appendix due to local gangrene may not cause the patient to lie up so long as local adhesions prevent the extension of the mischief. When the appendix ruptures into the general abdominal cavity in the absence of any protective adhesion, or when after being localized the inflammatory process extends, not even the most stoical or insensitive patient can refrain from seeking advice and taking to bed.

Obstruction of the lumen of the appendix, either by a concretion, stricture, kink, or adhesion, is usually accompanied by more acute and severe symptoms. So definite is the difference that some describe two forms of the disease—acute appendicitis and **acute appendical obstruction.** So far as this differentiation tends to emphasize the usually greater urgency of symptoms with obstruction of the lumen of the appendix it serves a useful purpose, but to treat the obstructive form as a different disease is quite unnecessary.

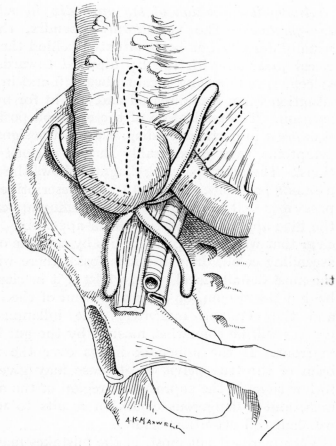

Fig. 10.—Diagram to show the various possible positions of the appendix vermiformis.

When the appendix has ruptured the pathological condition is not merely appendicitis, but peritonitis —local, diffuse, or general as the case may be—and diagnosis is to that extent more complicated. It is frequently only by careful attention to the history that one can make certain as to the true cause of such peritonitis.

Anatomical position of the appendix in relation to symptoms.—The vermiform appendix, though usually described as being situated behind the ileo-cæcal junction with the tip directed towards the spleen, is not by any means always found in that situation when it is diseased and sought for by the surgeon. The realization of the common positions is of great importance in diagnosis, for the signs and symptoms vary considerably in the various positions. The accompanying diagram shows the more common positions. (Fig. 10.) For descriptive purposes it is well to recognize the **ascending** appendix, the **iliac** appendix, and the **pelvic** appendix. It is clear that when the appendix lies by the side of the ascending colon, or in the iliac fossa, there will be the most definite local signs, whilst if it be situated behind the cæcum, or behind the end of the ileum and the common mesentery, the inflammatory process will be somewhat masked by the gut lying in front. If the appendix hangs over the right brim of the true pelvis the disease may give rise to few signs in the supra-pubic region of the abdomen, and a dangerous condition results to which we shall call attention below.

Very many, if not most, of the mistakes made in the diagnosis of appendicitis are due to a failure to realize the very great difference in signs and symptoms which follow from the varying position and relations of the appendix.

DIAGNOSIS OF APPENDICITIS BEFORE PERFORATION HAS TAKEN PLACE [1]

In any case of suspected appendicitis one must consider carefully :

(*A*) The history immediately prior to the onset of pain.

(*B*) The symptoms of the attack and the local signs.

(*C*) The order of occurrence of the symptoms.

The local conditions are more variable and notable after perforation has taken place, but there are definite indications even before perforation.

(*A*) There is frequently a *history* of indigestion, " gastritis," or flatulence for a few days prior to the onset of the attack. In a patient who has never, cr seldom, been subject to pain after taking food, this history should be sufficient to put one on guard. It may be elicited that frequent slight attacks of pain have been experienced in the appendicular region.

A history of unusual irregularity of the bowels is often obtained. Sometimes there is constipation, at other times diarrhœa, especially in children. The occurrence of diarrhœa is likely to mislead. It is probably due to the activity in the cæcum and colon of the virulent microbes which cause such damage to the appendix. In some cases an inflamed pelvic appendix may irritate the rectum. The early diarrhœa has to be distinguished from the late variety due to irritation of the rectum by pelvic peritonitis or a pelvic abscess.

[1] *Vide* Z. Cope, " The Preperitonitic Stage of Acute Appendicitis," *Brit. Med. Journ..* 1914.

(*B*) *The symptoms and local signs of the attack.*—
The signs and symptoms are :

> Pain (epigastric, then right iliac).
> Vomiting—nausea—acute loss of appetite.
> Local deep tenderness (per abdomen or per
>   rectum).
> Local rigidity of muscles (inconstant).
> Local distension (inconstant).
> Superficial hyperæsthesia (inconstant).
> Fever.
> Constipation.
> Testicular symptoms (uncommon).

Pain.—The pain in the majority of cases is first
referred to the epigastric or umbilical region, and
only later is localized in the right iliac fossa. Occasionally the initial pain is felt " all over the abdomen," though that is more usual in cases with perforation. Sometimes the pain is from the first hypogastric. When the appendix is retrocæcal in position
the initial pain may be felt in the right iliac region.
Though, therefore, the pain commonly starts in the
upper part of the abdomen, this is not invariable.

The causes of the early pain are probably two.
First and most important is the exaggerated
peristalsis of the appendix, excited by the relative
or absolute obstruction to its lumen by a concretion,
kink, or swollen mucous membrane ; bacterial
infection causes the accumulation of irritating
products which leads to a distension of the appendical lumen. Secondly, the upper abdominal pain
may sometimes be due to reflex pyloric spasm.

The epigastric pain is most acute and distinct in

those cases where there is considerable obstruction to the appendical lumen. *The localization of the pain to the right iliac region usually takes place some hours after the onset of the diffuse pain in the epigastric or umbilical regions.*

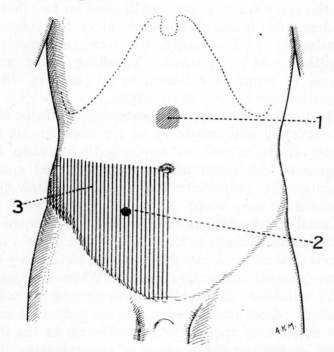

Fig. 11.—Diagram to show (1) common position of initial referred pain; (2) position of deep tenderness (nearly always to be elicited when abdominal wall not rigid); (3) shaded area to mark out the iliac triangle of hyperæsthesia in many cases of appendicitis.

Vomiting—Nausea—Anorexia. — Vomiting generally occurs in the early stages of the attack, but usually a few hours after the initial pain. Many patients do not vomit, but instead have a sensation of nausea. Loss of appetite or repulsion for food may be regarded as a lesser degree of the same sensation and often of equal value in diagnosis. Anyone in previously good health who suddenly develops anorexia and complains of abdominal pain should be carefully watched for appendicitis. The degree of nausea and the frequency of vomiting in the early stages appear to depend on two factors —first, the amount of distension of the inflamed appendix; and secondly, the reflex nervous susceptibility of the patient. Vomiting is the more prone to occur in children, or in patients whose digestive tract is easily deranged.

It may be taken as an important general rule that the severity and frequency of the vomiting at the onset of an attack of appendicitis indicate the degree of distension of the appendix and consequently the immediate risk to the patient that perforation may occur.

Local deep tenderness over the site of the appendix is frequently absent at the onset of the attack, and for some time the local symptoms are masked by the more general abdominal pains. When the latter have subsided the local deep tenderness is easily elicited. Occasionally even careful palpation cannot detect any spot of local tenderness in the iliac fossa during the *initial* stage of appendicitis. The place where deep tenderness can almost always be detected is a spot just below the middle of a line joining the anterior superior iliac spine and the umbilicus. This roughly corresponds to the position of the base of the appendix. Tenderness over MacBurney's spot is not so constant. This tenderness appears to be located actually in the appendix itself, for the site of the pain on pressure varies somewhat according to the position of the appendix, and is

obtainable when that viscus is not adherent to
any surrounding part. Sometimes the tenderness
may be due to adjacent peritoneal irritation. The
spot of maximum tenderness may sometimes be
accurately located by gentle percussion over the
affected region. In the case of an appendix situated
in the pelvis a rectal examination will frequently
elicit pain on pressing on the inflamed organ.

Local hyperæsthesia of the skin of the abdominal
wall is a frequent, but not a constant, accompaniment of an inflamed unperforated appendix. It
can be demonstrated in over half the cases of
appendicitis. Though occasionally bilateral, it is
usually confined to the right side. The areas
affected nearly always lie in the area of distribution
of the nerves from the tenth, eleventh, and twelfth
dorsal and first lumbar spinal segments. Though occasionally a zone of hyperæsthesia may be found
extending from the middle line in front back to the
spine, yet as a rule only the anterior part of the
abdominal wall is affected. Sometimes the right iliac
" appendix triangle " (Sherren) is demonstrable, at
other times only a part of such triangle is hyperæsthetic. (See Fig. 12.) As Sherren has pointed out,
hyperæsthesia depends largely on the degree of distension of the appendix. A common place in which
it can be elicited is a circumscribed area just to the
right of and on a level with the umbilicus. Sometimes the sensitive area is slightly lower than this,
but generally it lies in the area of distribution of the
tenth and eleventh thoracic spinal segments. When
there has been any local peritonitis in the iliac fossa
one can frequently elicit a band of hyperæsthesia immediately above and parallel to Poupart's ligament.

Local muscular rigidity over the inflamed area is frequently present, but is by no means a constant symptom in the initial stages. There are several

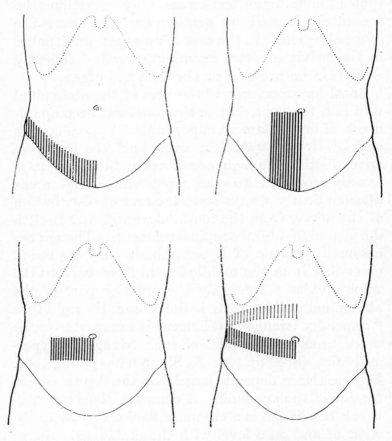

Fig. 12.—Types of hyperæsthesia (to pin stroke) which may be found in cases of acute and subacute appendicitis.

grades of muscular rigidity. The extreme degree is that in which the particular section of the abdominal wall is persistently stiff and will not move on respiration, in a lesser degree the muscle stiffens almost as soon as the hand touches the skin, and in the least degree the rigidity occurs only (and that to a slighter degree) when the fingers are pressed more deeply into the iliac fossa or towards the appendix. In most cases extreme muscular rigidity coincides with commencing peritonitis, and even slight degrees, when persisting, are due to irritation of the parietal peritoneum. It is a common experience to find no local muscular rigidity in a case of appendicitis without any peritonitis. In making this statement it must be understood that great care should be taken to exclude the rigidity which many patients develop as a result of nervousness and apprehension, or which may be induced by a rough or cold examining hand. Certainly with an unperforated appendix situated in the pelvis rigidity of the abdominal wall is nearly always absent. Failure to realize this important fact is responsible for many delayed operations and lost lives. *An appendix may be on the point of bursting into the general peritoneal cavity without a single adhesion to limit infection, though at the same time the abdominal wall may be flaccid and allow a free manipulation without any rigidity appearing.* This fact must be known to every surgeon of experience, but in general it is certainly not fully appreciated, nor do the textbooks make the point clear. Rigidity is taught to be one of the earliest signs of acute inflammation of the appendix, whereas in quite a large proportion of cases it is almost completely absent in the earliest stage, and in some cases is absent even though pelvic peritonitis exists.

When the inflammation of the appendix has caused œdema of the contiguous portions of the abdominal parietes (whether posterior, lateral, or anterior) muscular rigidity is the rule.

Rigidity of the psoas should always be tested for by extending the right thigh with the patient on the left side. Rigidity of the quadratus lumborum should be present with an inflamed ascending appendix. It is difficult to ascertain, but may be surmised if deep resistance be felt on pressing the fingers forward from beneath the lower posterior costal margin.

Fever may not be present at the beginning of the attack, but nearly always develops before twenty-four hours have passed. Before rupture has occurred the temperature does not usually go much above normal, two or three degrees Fahrenheit being the average elevation. Mistakes are liable to be made owing to the fact that the temperature is not elevated at the time of the onset of the pain, and thus the more serious disease may be mistaken for an attack of simple intestinal colic. In any suspected case the temperature should be taken every two or four hours, and if it rise in a gradual manner it is a point in favour of appendicitis. If at the very beginning of any attack of acute abdominal pain the temperature is considerably raised (i.e. 103° F. or 104° F.), the presumption is against appendicitis. Very rarely the illness may start with a rigor.

Though the patient frequently complains of constipation, yet numerous cases occur in which an attack of diarrhœa ushers in the attack.

The pulse is only slightly, if at all, accelerated in the early stage ; it may be normal in every way, even though the temperature be raised. *Any continued or decided acceleration of the pulse either corresponds with the occurrence of local peritonitis or indicates an appendix distended with infective material ;* to wait for such alteration is therefore to sacrifice the best time for operation.

When the appendix is acutely inflamed *gaseous distension of the cæcum* is frequently present ; this *local distension* is due partly to the excessive formation of gases by the active bacterial decomposition of the contents of the cæcum and appendix, and probably in some cases partly to an accompanying inflammation of the interior of the cæcum (typhlitis) with atony of the gut. It is more likely to be present when the appendix is retrocæcal in position and closely embedded in the wall of the cæcum. It gives rise to a local swelling with a tympanitic note on percussion, to borborygmi, and occasionally to painful peristaltic waves. This may cause the observer to think that he is merely dealing with a case of cæcal dyspepsia, and the swelling of the cæcum may mask the inflamed appendix placed behind it ; or the painful contractions of the distended gut attempting to empty itself may even suggest intestinal obstruction.

In the male, testicular symptoms are sometimes produced by an inflamed appendix even when unperforated. There may be pain in either right or left testicle, or in both, or the patient may say that the right testicle was retracted at a certain stage of the disease. The pain may possibly be due to irritation of the sympathetic filaments accompanying the spermatic artery, but it is more likely that it is a pain truly referred from the appendix since the tenth dorsal spinal segment apparently supplies both viscera. The direct stimulation of the genito-crural nerve by inflammatory exudate might account for testicular retraction.

(C) *The order of occurrence of the symptoms.*—This is of utmost importance in diagnosis. It is largely due to Murphy that the significance of the sequence of symptoms has been realized. The march of events is :

(1) Pain, usually epigastric or umbilical.
(2) Nausea or vomiting.
(3) Local iliac tenderness.
(4) Fever.
(5) Leucocytosis.

Murphy stated : " The symptoms occur almost without exception in the above order, and when that order varies I always question the diagnosis." Everyone who has carefully investigated the point must be able to confirm this dictum, though it must be allowed that occasional exceptions occur. If fever precedes the onset of pain, if vomiting accompanies or precedes the first bout of pain, it is generally not appendicitis with which we are dealing.

It is a fact worthy of remembrance that an acute attack of appendicitis often starts in the middle of the night, and may awaken the patient out of sleep.

There are two or three facts about the retrocæcal appendix that need special mention. Pain is usually less, and is often from the first felt only locally. Vomiting is not so frequent, and generally the muscular rigidity over the diseased focus is less than would be expected for so advanced a lesion.

The diagnosis of appendicitis in the stage prior

to perforation depends therefore upon certain constant and other inconstant features. Epigastric pain, nausea or vomiting, right iliac pain and fever in that symptom-sequence, are almost constant, and local tenderness, either on deep pressure in the right iliac region or by rectal examination, is invariable, except in the first hour or two of the attack. Local rigidity is common but not constant. The other symptoms mentioned above are inconstant, whilst the pulse-rate is usually normal and may mislead seriously.

In those rare cases in which, owing to developmental anomaly, the cæcum and appendix lie in the left instead of the right iliac fossa, the local symptoms and signs will be found on the left side. This condition is sometimes accompanied by dextrocardia, the existence of which should make one particularly careful in investigation of abdominal pain.

DIAGNOSIS AFTER PERFORATION HAS OCCURRED

It is to be regretted that so great a number of cases of acute appendicitis come to the surgeon after the appendix has perforated at the site of a patch of gangrene. One reason for this is that practitioners who send cases to surgeons are not always able to see the operations performed and consequently fail to realize that the symptoms of appendicitis as described in nearly all textbooks are those which accompany appendicitis with perforation of the appendix. It is the rule for practitioners to be surprised at the advanced state of the pathological process in cases where they thought they were advising an early operation. It is from those doctors who see their cases operated on that the early cases come. Local abscess means perforation of the appendix, and some estimate may thus be formed of the relative proportion of perforated and unperforated cases. In hospital practice probably the proportion of perforated and unperforated cases would be about equal. In private practice one obtains a larger proportion of unperforated cases. It must be allowed that in a few cases the first symptoms that the patient complains of seem to be those due to a perforation, but these cases are the exceptions.

The symptoms and course of illness consequent on appendicitis with perforation of the appendix are those already described, with the addition of the *symptoms due to local or diffuse peritonitis.* There are usually an accession of pain and renewal of vomiting when the perforation occurs, but the exact symptoms vary according to the position of the appendix and the nature of the protective peritoneal reaction.

Round the perforation itself a localized abscess may form, but sometimes a piece of omentum may seal the opening, or, more rarely, the infection may spread quickly and widely without the formation of any or many adhesions. A definite lump is generally though by no means always indicative of a perforation. In the absence of a perforation a lump may be caused by a thick and œdematous cæcum.

There are two main divisions of the pathological states consequent upon perforation depending upon the position of the appendix itself : (1) **when the appendix is above the brim of the true pelvis ;** (2) **when the appendix lies wholly or in part in the true pelvis.**

(1) **The iliac appendix.**—When an appendix lying above the pelvic brim ruptures there will be found on examination either a definite tender lump, a very definite rigidity of the abdominal wall over the site of the diseased viscus, or both rigidity and a lump.

In addition there will be fever (higher as a rule than before perforation), hyperæsthesia of the skin of the abdominal wall in the right iliac or right lumbar region, and certain localizing signs varying according to the position of the appendix.

(*a*) When the appendix perforates retrocæcally there will be a lump which may be resonant on percussion, owing to the intervening cæcum. The infection will cause inflammatory œdema of the iliacus and quadratus lumborum and adjacent parts, and tenderness will be elicited on pressing the fingers forward below the right costal margin at the outer border of the erector spinæ.

(*b*) The appendix may lie in a position parallel with the cæcum and ascending colon, but lateral to them. The symptoms are then similar to those just described, save that rigidity of the lateral and anterior abdominal wall is more evident, and that any lump is more easily felt because the cæcum does not mask it.

(*c*) The conditions resulting from perforation of an appendix lying in the iliac fossa on the iliacus or psoas are sufficiently characteristic. Immediately after the perforation there will be intense rigidity of the abdominal wall over the right iliac region and great tenderness on pressure over the same area. (Very rarely, chiefly in patients suffering from severe toxic absorption, rigidity which had at first been present disappears on perforation of the appendix.)

After a certain time, if suitable resistance be offered to the infection, the peritoneal reaction becomes limited, and the rigidity usually diminishes somewhat, allowing the palpating hand to feel a tender lump—either due to a small local abscess or a mass of omentum wrapped round the inflamed perforated appendix.

There are two special symptoms which may help exact localization in this region. The irritation and reflex rigidity of the ilio-psoas frequently cause the patient to hold the right thigh flexed, or with a lesser degree of irritation pain may be felt only if the right thigh be fully extended as the patient lies on the left side. This sign is often of great value.

In a few cases irritation of the external cutaneous nerve as it crosses the iliacus is evidenced by pain and hyperæsthesia along the distribution of that nerve.

(d) When the appendix lies so that the tip is directed medialwards the result of its perforation varies greatly according to whether it is behind or in front of the ileum. If *behind the ileum* localization of the inflammatory process usually results, but the swelling is not so readily felt since the ileum covers and masks it. But tenderness and rigidity may be present, and an indefinite lump may be felt, whilst the test for psoas-irritation may help in diagnosis.

The ureter crosses the pelvic brim in close relationship to the medially directed appendix, and occasionally pain on micturition may be produced presumably by irritation of the ureter.

If the appendix perforates whilst lying *in front of the ileum* there is great danger of very extensive peritonitis, but if the infection becomes localized diagnosis is fairly easy, for the formation of pus close up against the abdominal wall leads to local boardlike rigidity and exquisite tenderness (hyperalgesia) over the affected area. Psoas-irritation will be absent.

(2) **The pelvic appendix.**—The early symptoms of an attack of appendicitis when the appendix is situated in the pelvis are similar to those which ensue when it is situated above the pelvic brim, with the exception that rigidity of the right iliac region of the abdominal wall is seldom present in the early stages, and that the pain is more frequently felt in both left and right iliac fossæ. Pain is not so readily localized in the right iliac fossa, but is always felt on deep pressure at the brim of the true pelvis, and the epigastric pain may dominate the scene for a longer time.

The perforated pelvic appendix is one of the most easily overlooked, and therefore one of the most dangerous conditions which may occur in the abdomen. The reason appears to be as follows. Whilst the appendix is unruptured and tense the pain due to the distension and peristaltic contraction is definite and severe, and is felt chiefly in the epigastrium or umbilical zone. When rupture occurs the epigastric pain diminishes and local pelvic peritonitis results on the right side of the pelvis or at the bottom of the pelvic pouch of peritoneum. *This is usually unaccompanied by rigidity of the lower abdominal muscles,* and since the pain of appendicular distension has ceased, and the pain due to pelvic peritonitis at this stage is frequently very insignificant, the patient may seem better, and the examina-

tion of the abdomen may give little indication of
the trouble in the pelvis. Sooner or later—usually
within three or four days—the peritonitis either

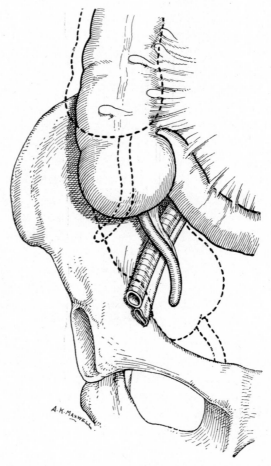

Fig. 13.— Diagram to show positions the cæcum may occupy.

becomes definitely localized into a pelvic abscess of
considerable dimensions, or the inflammation may
track upwards towards the general abdominal

cavity and give rise to increasing pain, distension, and rigidity of the abdominal wall. If from the fact that the patient came late for advice, or that sufficient attention was not paid to the preliminary symptoms and symptom-sequence, the pre-rupture stage of the inflamed pelvic appendix is missed, it is at least essential to diagnose the ruptured appendix as soon as possible after rupture before peritonitis has extended too far upwards into the abdominal cavity. For this purpose it is important to pay attention to the anatomical position of the pelvic appendix, which lies in relationship with one or more of the following—*the pelvic wall, the rectum, and the bladder.* Irritation of the bladder or rectum may be signified by frequency of or pain during micturition, or by diarrhœa or tenesmus respectively. But more important is the fact that usually a tender swelling can be felt against the right pelvic wall by the finger inserted into the rectum. Moreover, when the ruptured appendix is adherent to the fascia covering the obturator internus and the subjacent fibres of the muscle are affected by the inflammatory œdema, rotation of the flexed thigh so as to put the muscle through its extreme movements (especially internal rotation) will cause hypogastric pain. In performing this manœuvre it is essential that the thigh be flexed so as to relax the psoas muscle.

By a careful consideration of the history and of the points just mentioned it should be difficult to miss the early inflamed pelvic appendix. The appendix which is most likely to give rise to doubt in diagnosis is one situated high up in the right posterior quadrant of the pelvis, for in this situation there may be no localizing signs and it may be difficult to feel the viscus per rectum.

The later symptoms resulting from rupture of a pelvic appendix are either those of a large pelvic abscess or those of advanced pelvic and hypogastric peritonitis, with increasing toxæmia. Tenderness and rigidity of the whole lower abdominal wall, distension, vomiting, and increased pain, all give a clear picture of peritonitis.

It is noteworthy that as the peritonitic inflammation spreads upwards from the pelvis it does so frequently on the left side first. This is probably because as the pelvis fills with pus the anatomical path of least resistance is by the side of the sigmoid colon.

When a pelvic abscess has formed there are usually all the symptoms of suppuration—fever, furred tongue, anorexia, and leucocytosis, whilst locally there are tenderness and slight distension in the hypogastrium. Rigidity of the lower abdominal wall is quite frequently absent, even when a pelvic abscess is present. Occasionally the temperature may be normal even though an abscess be present.

Per rectum the bulge of the abscess can easily be detected, and pain is produced by pressing on the bulging mass.

In women the intervention of the uterus makes bladder-symptoms less likely to supervene in cases of appendicular suppuration. The normal uterine loss may be increased by the pelvic congestion and the menstrual period may be precipitated thereby.

There is a rare condition of intestinal obstruction which is said to be produced by pelvic appendicular suppuration at a late stage. Both the sigmoid colon and the small intestine may be obstructed within the pelvis. Mr. Handley has termed the condition ileus duplex. But if the inflamed pelvic appendix were diagnosed in the early stage there would never arise any such dangerous late complication. In early diagnosis and operation lies the prevention of such conditions.

CHAPTER V

THE DIFFERENTIAL DIAGNOSIS OF APPENDICITIS

DIAGNOSIS of appendicitis is usually easy. Considerably over 50 per cent. of the acute abdominal emergencies admitted to a hospital are cases of appendicular inflammation. So frequent is the condition that it would almost appear that some do not trouble to attempt a differential diagnosis, since many mistakes are made which might easily be avoided by a careful examination.

The typical case with epigastric pain, followed by vomiting, succeeded by localizing of the pain in the right iliac fossa where tenderness can always and rigidity of the overlying rectus can usually be made out, is sufficiently characteristic, even without the presence of slight fever, to make the diagnosis certain. But there are certain difficulties which need to be discussed.

It is important first to make quite sure that one is dealing with a primarily abdominal condition. In the course of a definite attack of **influenza** abdominal pain may ensue, and during an outbreak of the disease there is grave danger that occasionally an attack of appendicitis may be overlooked and attributed to " abdominal influenza." But seldom in influenza is the abdomen alone attacked, and a local examination will usually determine whether the site of the pain be appendicular. Yet pain and tenderness in the right iliac fossa are sometimes present in influenza, though the abdominal pain is more likely to be general, and borborygmi may sometimes be heard all over the abdomen. Backache and pain in the eyeballs are more likely to be felt in an attack of influenza and vomiting may precede the abdominal pain—a sequence seldom seen in appendicitis.

Again, one must always exclude **diaphragmatic pleurisy** or early basal pneumonia before diagnosing appendicitis. Pain, tenderness, and muscular rigidity may all be noted in the right iliac region in thoracic disease, but sometimes firm continued pressure will enable one to feel deep into the iliac fossa without causing any increase of the pain. In cases of appendicitis pressure over the left iliac fossa carried out by fingers pressed deeply in and directed towards the right side will sometimes cause pain in the appendicular region—a sign which is absent in cases of pleurisy or pneumonia. In thoracic disease the respiration-rate is usually increased, and the pulse-respiration ratio diminished. Of course, a careful examination of the chest is *the* method of discrimination.

Very rarely **spinal disease** may cause pain referred to the appendicular region. An examination of the spinal column can easily and quickly be made, and would soon determine any lesion. On one occasion I have known osteomyelitis of the ilium simulate acute appendicitis. In this case the boy looked very ill, had fever and local iliac pain, but there was no muscular rigidity.

Typhoid fever is another general disease which is occasionally mistaken for appendicitis, because of the abdominal pain and tenderness which are sometimes localized in the right iliac fossa. In most cases, however, there are general symptoms which would enable the diagnosis to be made. Headache, general malaise, enlargement of the spleen, presence of a roseola, and the absence of the acute onset so usual in appendicitis, should make one suspicious of typhoid, and the absence of a leucocytosis would exclude appendicitis. In children in whom the general symptoms of typhoid fever are often slight, and occasionally in adults attacked by the ambulatory type of the disease, mistakes might be made. In some doubtful cases the presence of definite cutaneous hyperæsthesia would decide in favour of appendicitis.

A true typhoid appendicitis is sometimes seen. I once operated on a lad who had typical symptoms of appendicitis, and removed an appendix crowded with thread-worms and having an ulcerated mucous membrane. The pathologist who examined the appendix stated that he had never previously seen ulceration caused by thread-worms alone. The child's temperature kept up in an irregular manner after operation, and an agglutination-test to the *bacillus typhosus* proved positive. This kind of case, in which the symptoms of a true typhoid appendicitis initiate the illness, is uncommon.

If the symptoms have been present for a week when the patient is first seen the agglutination-reaction may be positive in respect to *bacillus typhosus* (*Eberthella typhosa*) or *paratyphosus a* or *b*. A blood-culture of a typhoid patient might prove positive if taken within the first week of the disease. One must utter a warning against treating any doubtful case as typhoid without making a rectal examination. The irregular fever, tympanitic abdomen, and vague hypogastric pains which accompany a pelvic abscess may be and have been mistaken for typhoid fever, but a finger inserted into the anal canal will serve to distinguish.

In the stage of *catarrhal* appendicitis before there is any or much congestion or inflammation of the peritoneum, and when muscular rigidity is often if not usually absent, appendicitis is sometimes mistakenly diagnosed as :

Gastritis.
Indigestion.
A bilious attack.
Colic.

The fact that the initial pain is frequently felt in the epigastrium is responsible for the diagnosis of gastritis or indigestion. The sudden onset, often without any relationship to food-taking (e.g. in the middle of the night), together with the gradual localization of pain in the right iliac fossa, and the onset of slight fever, should give sufficient ground for a diagnosis. The danger is that with such slight symptoms the observer may not even make a thorough abdominal examination, or may omit a rectal examination whereby an inflamed pelvic appendix might be diagnosed.

When vomiting or nausea is a notable feature of the attack it is sometimes erroneously attributed to a *bilious attack*. This is especially the case with children, in whom such a diagnosis must always be carefully made, and only after appendicitis has been fully excluded. It is a common experience for the surgeon who has removed a gangrenous appendix from a child's abdomen to be told by the parents or practitioner that the child had always been subject to bilious attacks, for one of which attacks the acute illness had at first been mistaken. Any child, previously in good health, who is suddenly taken with abdominal pain and loss of appetite, has nausea, or vomits, and at the same time shows definite deep tenderness in the right iliac fossa, even if the pulse be normal and the temperature not elevated, is most probably suffering from appendicitis.

Before a diagnosis of *intestinal colic* be made appendicular colic must be excluded. If a few hours after the onset of the pain there still be no tenderness elicited on pressing over the right iliac fossa or right pelvic brim, and none on the right side of the pelvis (by rectal examination) it may fairly be excluded. In simple colic pressure on the painful part often relieves the pain.

When the local signs and symptoms of appendicitis are well developed (pain, tenderness, hyperæsthesia, rigidity) there are very many conditions which have to be excluded, and for which it may be mistaken. When the local signs are very clear the appendix is usually either perforated or in danger of perforating. To catalogue the diseases which *may* simulate or be simulated by appendicitis is to enumerate all the chief acute abdominal diseases. This is obviously of little practical value. It will be better, therefore, to give only the more common conditions causing mistakes and to group them according to the position of the appendix :

The ascending appendix (**Retrocæcal or Paracæcal**) :
Cholecystitis.
Inflamed duodenal ulcer.
Perforated gall-bladder.
Perinephric abscess.
Hydronephrosis.
Pyonephrosis.
Pyelitis.
Stone in the kidney.

Iliac position of appendix :
Leaking duodenal ulcer.
Cæcal or ileo-cæcal carcinoma.
Psoas abscess.
Ileo-cæcal tuberculosis.
Hip disease.
Tuberculous ileo-cæcal glands.
Stone in the ureter.
Crohn's disease (Regional enteritis).

Pelvic position of appendix :
Intestinal obstruction.
Diverticulitis with abscess.
Perforation of a typhoid ulcer.

In women :
Ectopic gestation.
Twisted pedicle of an ovarian cyst or of a hydrosalpinx.
Rupture of a pyosalpinx.
Salpingitis.

Before diagnosing appendicitis in tropical climes one would also have to exclude :

Amœbic typhlitis.

Hepatitis.

Leaking liver-abscess.

Malaria.

When the local manifestations have spread widely and the patient first comes under observation with generalized peritonitis, it is necessary to distinguish the condition from all the various causes which may lead to such a pathological picture.

Late cases with extensive peritonitis must be distinguished from :

Acute intestinal obstruction. (See
    Chapter VII.)
Thrombosis or embolism of mesenteric
    vessels. (See p. 135.)
Acute pancreatitis. (See p. 114.)
Pneumococcal peritonitis. (See p. 240.)
Pylephlebitis.
General peritonitis (ruptured gastric,
    duodenal, typhoid ulcers, etc.).

DIFFERENTIAL DIAGNOSIS OF THE PERFORATING OR PERFORATED ASCENDING APPENDIX

The gall-bladder, the duodenum, and the kidney are the viscera in anatomical proximity to the ascending appendix, and inflammation of them or their surroundings may cause difficulty in diagnosis.

Cholecystitis may very closely simulate appendicitis. Pain, vomiting, fever, constipation, and local tenderness on the right side of the abdomen are present in both cases. An enlarged inflamed gall-bladder frequently comes down into the right lumbar region, but more usually enlarges in the direction of the umbilicus. In thin subjects without rigidity of the abdominal wall diagnosis is usually easy, for the tender rounded gall-bladder may be felt continuous with the liver and perhaps moving with respiration. The pain in cholecystitis is usually a little higher than that of an ascending appendicitis, and there may be pain of a segmental nature referred to the right subscapular region, especially if a stone be impacted in the cystic duct. There may be resonance of the ascending colon over an inflamed retrocæcal appendix. There is never resonance in front of an inflamed gall-bladder, which is usually on an anterior plane to the cæcum, colon, and appendix. In very stout subjects and in patients with very rigid abdominal muscles it may on occasion be almost impossible to diagnose whether the appendix or gall-bladder be at fault without giving an anæsthetic, unless the previous history be clearly indicative of one or other condition.

When with the cholecystitis a stone is simultaneously impacted in the cystic duct the constant spasms of pain accompanied by retching, with deep tenderness in the right hypochondrium and right subscapular region, are sufficiently diagnostic and clearly differentiated from appendicitis.

Periduodenitis round an inflamed duodenal ulcer should be distinguishable by the characteristic history elicited by careful questioning. The pain of duodenal ulcer comes two or three hours after food, and is relieved by the taking of food.

Acute right-sided pyelitis is frequently mistaken for appendicitis, and not infrequently operations are unwisely undertaken because insufficient attention is paid to the symptoms. The points in differential diagnosis can be tabulated as follows :

ACUTE PYELITIS.	APPENDICITIS.
Initial rigor common.	Rigor unusual.
Temperature 103° or more.	Temperature so high as 103° uncommon.
Pain on micturition.	
Increased frequency of urination.	Urinary symptoms inconstant.
Abdominal muscles often lax.	Local rigidity frequent.
Pus or bacteria in urine.	No pus in urine.

The symptoms of acute pyelitis may be produced by the presence of bacilli in the urine without any or much formation of pus. In such cases there is always a turbidity or opalescence of the urine which is suggestive of the bacilluria. One must not forget also that an inflamed appendix lying in front of the renal pelvis may actually cause an acute pyelitis.

If the urine be carefully examined as a routine there will seldom be any difficulty in diagnosis.

Acute right-sided hydronephrosis is sometimes misdiagnosed appendicitis with abscess formation. A hydronephrosis forms a rounded, tense, tender swelling which occupies the lateral aspect of the abdomen and can be felt well back in the loin. The swelling is sometimes freely movable and usually rounded in shape. It may be possible to feel a depression (corresponding with the hilum) on the medial side. The pain is sometimes of the type of renal colic and *there are usually urinary symptoms*—scanty urine, pain during or frequency of micturition, etc. It may be possible to ascertain a history of previous attacks corresponding to Dietl's crises. Rigidity of the abdominal wall over the swelling is usually absent.

Acute pyonephrosis forms a similar swelling to a hydronephrosis, but it is usually more tender, more fixed, and the general signs of constitutional disturbance are much greater, e.g. there are high fever, very furred tongue, and maybe other symptoms of toxæmia. There may be pus in the urine.

Movable kidney *without hydronephrosis.*—A kinking of the reno-ureteric junction may occur and cause severe pain in the loin and diminution of amount of urinary secretion, without much swelling of the kidney. The urinary symptoms, lack of fever, and relief of the pain when urine passes more freely, serve to distinguish.

Stone in the kidney or ureter.—In those unusual cases in which appendicitis is accompanied by pain in the right testis it may closely simulate renal colic. An X-ray photograph should show the stone and differentiate. Cases do occur, however, in which small ureteric calculi do not show on an X-ray negative, and then the character of the pain must be the deciding factor in diagnosis. In one case under my care acute pain in the right loin radiating to the right testis, accompanied by fever and some muscular rigidity, caused me to diagnose renal colic. A radiograph showed a large shadow a little external to the normal line of the ureter. Operation revealed a normal kidney and ureter, but a very inflamed appendix with a large calcareous gland in the meso-appendix. Fortunately such cases are rare.

Torsion of omentum.—Torsion and strangulation of a portion of omentum may simulate appendicitis. The part affected is usually to the right of the midline, and pain and tenderness will be noted to the right of the umbilicus. If the affected fat becomes adherent to the abdominal wall there may be superficial hyperæsthesia. Vomiting is less common than in appendicitis, but differential diagnosis before operation may be impossible.

Perinephric abscess.—A suppurating retrocæcal appendix may form an abscess in the neighbourhood of the kidney, and may be difficult to diagnose from a perinephric abscess of metastatic origin. But the latter is insidious in origin, whilst appendicitis usually gives a typically acute history of onset. In both cases there will be pain on pressing forward in the erector-costal angle below the last rib. Some patients with an inflamed retrocæcal appendix present atypical symptoms, have no initial epigastric pain, do not vomit, and present no rigidity over the inflamed area. *These cases, however, are much more rapid in development than the usual metastatic perinephric abscess.* A small retrocæcal or retro-ileal abscess of appendicular origin may easily be overlooked. (See Fig. 14.)

DIFFERENTIAL DIAGNOSIS OF THE INFLAMED ILIAC APPENDIX

Inflammation of the iliac appendix is the most easy to diagnose, though there are many pitfalls.

A perforated duodenal ulcer is frequently mis-diagnosed appendicitis. The escaping contents travel down first to the iliac fossa and give rise to all the signs of inflammation of the appendix. It may be possible to obtain a typical duodenal or appendicular history. The initial shock at onset is greater in the duodenal condition, and there will also be definite right hypochondriac tenderness. Pain felt on the top of the right shoulder would be more in favour of a perforated duodenal ulcer. If there be any obliteration of liver-dullness in the absence of general abdominal distension a duodenal (or gastric) perforation is certain.

Carcinoma or tuberculosis of the ileo-cæcal junction.—When a carcinoma or hyperplastic tuberculosis causes any obstruction at the ileo-cæcal valve appendicitis may readily be simulated. There will be recurring attacks of severe pain, vomiting, local distension and tenderness in the right iliac fossa, and sometimes rigidity during or after the attack. But the pain in ileo-cæcal obstruction is more griping and intense than in appendicitis, and the vomiting comes on almost simultaneously with the pain, and is more violent and persistent than in any but the most advanced appendicular peritonitis. Sooner or later an attack of complete obstruction will occur and general distension ensue. Constipation is noticed during the attacks, and loss of weight rapidly takes place.

Carcinoma of the cæcum *or ascending colon* which forms a tumour, and which has become adherent to the parietes, or which has eroded the gut and caused a perityphlitic abscess, may simulate an abscess of appendicular origin. The age of the patient (usually over fifty), previous attacks suggestive of obstruction, noticeable loss of weight and anæmia, usually help to distinguish, but cases do occur in which differential diagnosis is almost impossible before operation.

Ileo-cæcal tuberculosis of the non-obstructive type may cause symptoms similar to those of carcinoma, and indeed may not be distinguishable prior to operation.

Tuberculous ileo-cæcal glands are easily mistaken for an inflamed appendix. They occur chiefly in children, and cause slight tenderness, and maybe a lump, in the right iliac fossa. If the glands are fleshy and tending to undergo caseation they may cause inflammation of the contiguous mesentery and peritoneum, and the local signs will be increased by the presence of greater local tenderness and possibly muscular rigidity. Nausea or vomiting may occur, but epigastric pain is not so likely to be in evidence, and the typical symptom-sequence will not be obtained. Tuberculous mesenteric glands may be accompanied by an irregular fever. An X-ray photo may show some calcification in the glands.

Psoas abscess and *tuberculous hip disease* may each cause irritation of the ilio-psoas with flexion or limitation of extension of the right thigh, and tenderness, resistance, and fullness in the right iliac fossa, but the general onset and subacute nature of the illness, together with careful examination of the spine and hip, in most cases easily establish the diagnosis. A radiograph should be taken if doubt exists.

Stone in the ureter.—A stone passing down the ureter causes pain, not always typical of renal colic, referred approximately to that section of the ureter in which the stone is lodged. Quite frequently this causes a diagnosis of appendicitis to be made. Urinary symptoms (frequency, pain, hæmaturia), pain in the testicle, absence of rigidity over the painful area, and a previous history of attacks suggestive of renal colic, should put one on to the right line of diagnosis ; and if expert assistance be available, radiography and cystoscopy with the passage up the ureter of the affected side of a wax-tipped bougie may serve to demonstrate a calculus. Fever is unlikely to be present in the case of ureteral stone.

An abscess developing in the abdominal wall in the right iliac region may be difficult to diagnose from appendicitis, but the history, absence of vomiting, and superficial localization without any deep signs, should differentiate.

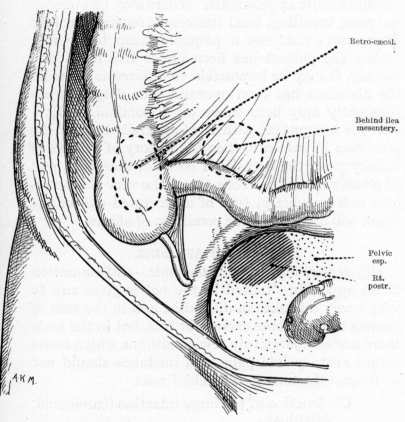

Fig. 14.—Diagram showing those sites where an abscess resulting from appendicitis may sometimes be overlooked.   (See pages 86 and 93.)

Rupture of the lower segment of the right rectus muscle may also lead to local signs similar to those caused by appendicitis, but the history of onset should serve to distinguish. Rupture of the rectus is prone to follow a great or sudden muscular effort, or may be due to a severe bout of coughing. Vomiting and intestinal symptoms will be absent.

Crohn's disease or **Regional enteritis** may closely simulate acute appendicitis. There may be abdominal pain, vomiting, local tenderness in the right iliac fossa, and sometimes a palpable lump to be felt. Unless the patient has been under treatment previously, it may be impossible to differentiate before the abdomen has been opened. The diagnosis has frequently only been made on abdominal exploration for a supposed attack of appendicitis. If the condition be subacute then the history of attacks of colicky pain, the occasional bouts of diarrhoea, and (if a barium meal has been given) the very characteristic radiographic picture of a narrowed end of the ileum will reveal the true condition of affairs.

THE PELVIC APPENDIX

Differential diagnosis in the male.—Inflammation of an appendix situated in the pelvis gives rise to very many mistakes in diagnosis, and in the case of women there is some excuse for this, but in the male there are comparatively few conditions which cause severe acute pelvic pain, and mistakes should not so frequently occur. The chief are :

> Obstruction of the large intestine (carcinoma, volvulus).
> Obstruction of the small intestine.
> Diverticulitis.
> Stone in the lower part of the ureter.

Obstruction of the large bowel causing hypogastric symptoms is commonly due to carcinoma of the sigmoid or rectum, or to volvulus. The onset of both these conditions is usually preluded by a time of subacute obstruction with attacks of abdominal pain and distension, and in both cases *distension is an early feature of the acute attack.* In pelvic appendicitis the symptom-sequence is fairly constant, and *distension is not* an early symptom. In both cases rectal examination will reveal pelvic tenderness, but in obstruction there may be greater ballooning of the upper part of the rectum, whilst in appendicitis there is often a tender lump on the right side of the pelvis, and the thigh-rotation test may be positive. In appendicitis also there is not complete obstruction, and a turpentine enema will bring away flatus and fæcal material. Fever is usually absent in obstruction, and present in appendicitis.

Obstruction of the ileum, accompanied by tenderness in the hypogastrium, is frequently due to adhesions caused by former attacks of appendicitis. The adhesions usually bind the end of the ileum down to the lateral wall of the pelvis or the bottom of the pelvic pouch of peritoneum. The previous history of appendicitis may deceive. Distinction is to be made chiefly by noting that in obstruction there is greater acuteness of pain, which is of a spasmodic nature, and by observing the frequency and character of the vomit, which in obstruction gradually becomes yellowish and finally fæculent— a change which never happens in appendicitis until extensive peritonitis has developed. In intestinal obstruction the pain is seldom localized in the right iliac fossa as in appendicitis, but after distension has supervened diagnosis is made much more difficult. In small-bowel obstruction also the temperature is usually subnormal at onset, and does not at any period become febrile as is usual in appendicitis. Frequency of micturition or pain during the act may occur in appendicitis, owing to irritation of the bladder.

Diverticulitis of the pelvic colon may cause either obstructive or inflammatory symptoms. When causing obstruction it closely resembles carcinoma, but when local inflammation and abscess result the symptoms and signs are very similar to those of pelvic appendicitis, and there is no certain way of distinguishing before operation since in these cases a barium enema is inadvisable. Diverticulitis is, however, a condition chiefly met with in older persons, and there may be a history of previous bowel derangement which may be referable to the colon, e.g. attacks of diarrhœa and constipation, or passage of slime and blood, etc. The *initial* pain is more likely to be hypogastric in pelvic pericolitis and epigastric in appendicitis.

Perforation of a typhoid ulcer.—When, in a patient suffering from a mild attack of typhoid fever, a subacute perforation occurs in the lower ileum, a pelvic abscess may result which may at the time of examination be indistinguishable clinically from that due to a perforated appendix. But the diagnosis will be helped by the previous history. In one case which came under my care the patient had been treated for two weeks for influenza before the pelvic symptoms caused her to be sent up to hospital for appendicitis. A pelvic abscess was opened, and a blood agglutination test proved that *B. paratyphosus a* (*Salmonella paratyphi*) was the cause of the disease.

Stone in the lower part of the ureter (see p. 90).—
When a stone is near the bladder there are often
additional symptoms, frequency, strangury, pain
in the penis, emissions, which may point to the
genito-urinary system. Cystoscopy might show
a pouting right ureteric orifice, and a catheter put
up the ureter would stop at the site of the stone.

A *Pelvic Abscess* following appendicitis is frequently overlooked especially when occupying the
right posterior quadrant of pelvis (Fig. 14).

DIFFERENTIAL DIAGNOSIS OF PELVIC APPENDICITIS IN THE FEMALE

The female reproductive organs add considerably
to the difficulty in diagnosis of pelvic appendicitis.
Acute pain referable specially to the hypogastrium
and pelvis may be due to :

> Uterine colic (dysmenorrhœa or threatening
> abortion).
> Twisted pedicle, inflammation, or rupture of
> an ovarian cyst, or torsion of a normal
> or slightly enlarged ovary.
> Ectopic gestation.
> Twisted or inflamed fibroid.
> Twisted hydrosalpinx.
> Salpingitis or pyosalpinx.
> Rupture of an endometrioma.

Dysmenorrhœa, with its periodicity, lack of signs
on local examination, and pain referred to the lower
lumbar and sacral region as well as the hypogastrium,
should not cause serious difficulty in diagnosis.

In **threatened abortion,** the previous amenorrhœa,
bleeding, character of the pain, and absence of local
signs easily serve to distinguish.

Ectopic gestation is frequently misdiagnosed appendicitis, but there is usually some menstrual irregularity, often a history of a fainting attack, general anæmia, and a displaced uterus, whilst the symptom-sequence of appendicitis is not usually seen. In unruptured cases the enlarged tube may be felt as an abnormal mobile and tender swelling to one side of the uterus. (See Chapter XII.)

In the case of an **ovarian cyst or hydrosalpinx, with a twisted pedicle,** diagnosis is made chiefly by the fact that with the twisted viscus *the pain and vomiting come on simultaneously* (or almost so), so that the proper appendix symptom-sequence is wanting; moreover the vomiting or retching is usually more frequent and more persistent than in appendicitis. In the case of an ovarian cyst it may have been previously known that there was a tumour, and a definite tender swelling may be made out from the time of onset of the symptoms. This swelling may be situated in the mid-hypogastrium or to one or other side, or may be limited to the pelvis. Superficial hyperæsthesia to pin-stroke in the right iliac region is commonly found with appendicitis, but is less frequently detected with an ovarian cyst. Torsion of a normal ovary may occur. If this happens in early pregnancy there may be difficulty in distinguishing it from an early ectopic pregnancy or a pelvic appendicitis.

With a twisted fibroid the symptoms are not usually so acute, and the presence of the fibroid will most likely have been known previously. It may be impossible to differentiate between twisted fibroid and an ovarian cyst with twisted pedicle.

Acute salpingitis is frequently difficult to distinguish from appendicitis, and sometimes the two occur simultaneously. Occasionally it is difficult to say in which of the contiguous organs the inflammation started. Distinction may usually be made by considering the following points. Acute salpingitis does not so frequently cause epigastric pain at the onset, and vomiting is less frequent. The salpingitic pain is frequently felt on both sides from the onset and there may be greater tenderness in the left iliac region than the right. The history is often unreliable, but the presence of a vaginal discharge is a valuable guide and examination should be directed to this point. It has been stated that with salpingitis pain is more often felt down the thigh even as far as the knee, but this is certainly not a constant symptom. If in doubt, it is better that operation should be undertaken, but if there is no reasonable doubt that the condition is acute salpingitis there are many surgeons who consider non-operative treatment, by putting the patient into the Fowler position and giving rectal saline injections, quite satisfactory. The advent of penicillin, to which the gonococcus is sensitive, has made operative treatment of acute gonococcal salpingitis unnecessary.

A **pyosalpinx** may rupture and cause simulation of a pelvic appendicitis. The typical appendicular symptom-sequence is usually wanting. If examination be made soon after the onset of symptoms a pelvic swelling will be felt. This is usually bilateral. A history of chronic pelvic pain and leucorrhœa may be ascertained. In cases coming under observation after some days diagnosis may be impossible before operation.

Rupture of an ovarian endometrioma may closely simulate a pelvic appendicitis. Sudden hypogastric pain, vomiting, slight fever, and tenderness on pelvic examination may be present in both cases, but with an endometrioma a unilateral or bilateral swelling ought to be detected on bimanual examination.

In late cases of appendicitis which have led to a very diffuse or general peritonitis, or in those cases of a very fulminating type which are associated with a rapid form of spreading peritonitis, it is often impossible to make a certain diagnosis. Distinction has to be made from :

> Primary pneumococcal peritonitis.
> Secondary general peritonitis due to other causes (rupture of gastric, duodenal, typhoid, stercoral, or carcinomatous ulcer, or of a pyosalpinx).
> Thrombosis of mesenteric vessels.
> Acute intestinal obstruction.
> Acute pancreatitis.
> Pylephlebitis.

In finding out the exact cause the greatest importance attaches to the history. The subject is considered more fully in the next chapter and in that on peritonitis.

CHAPTER VI

PERFORATION OF A GASTRIC OR DUODENAL ULCER

(A) Perforation into the General Peritoneal Cavity

Perforation of a gastric or duodenal ulcer into the general peritoneal cavity is a catastrophe which occurs with dramatic suddenness, and unless treated surgically progresses in a definite manner with a typical course until the death of the patient about two or three days after the perforation. It is one of the most easily diagnosed acute abdominal conditions, provided the symptoms are known and appreciated, and it is the most important to diagnose early and treat promptly by surgical intervention. We say this advisedly, although we are aware that some cases have been and may be treated successfully without operation. Delay in the diagnosis of appendicitis is regrettable, but does not always cost the patient's life. Misdiagnosis of an inflamed gallbladder or a pyosalpinx is a perilous occurrence, but the position may frequently be retrieved by a later operation; but in the case of a perforated ulcer a delayed diagnosis, or a misdiagnosis which leads to temporizing and delay, is equivalent to a death sentence with very slight chance of reprieve. If operation be undertaken within the first six hours recovery is the rule, if the opening of the abdomen be delayed for twelve hours recovery is more doubt-ful, if twenty-four or more hours elapse prior to suture of the ulcer and drainage of the abdomen the death of the patient is to be expected. True, some cases recover though operated on at a later stage than this, but they are always regarded as exceptional and worthy of comment. The very possibility of any condition being due to a perforated ulcer is a positive indication for an *immediate* solution of the problem. If the problem cannot be solved with certainty, action should be taken for removal of the patient to the nearest surgical centre. To leave the diagnosis in doubt overnight will most likely cost the patient's life if a perforation be present.

The signs and symptoms produced by the per-foration vary according to the time which has elapsed since the rupture occurred. There are three stages in the pathological process which can usually be recognized easily :

(1) The stage of prostration or primary shock.
(2) The stage of reaction (with masked peri-tonitis).
(3) The stage of (advanced) frank peritonitis and secondary or toxic shock.

There is no hard-and-fast limit between the stages, and occasionally primary shock may lead on to frank peritonitis and terminal collapse without any noticeable interval of reaction.

The symptoms of each stage can be enumerated :

Stage of prostration or primary shock:
Great and generalized abdominal pain.
Anxious countenance.
Livid or ashen appearance.

Stage of prostration or primary shock (*continued*) :
    Cold extremities.
    Cold sweating face.
    Subnormal temperature (95° or 96° F.).
    Pulse small and weak.
    Shallow respiration.
    Retching or vomiting.
    Pain on the top of one or both shoulders.

Stage of reaction (masked peritonitis) :
    Vomiting ceases.
    Abdominal pain less.
    Appearance much better, face regains normal colour.
    Temperature normal.
    Pulse normal.
    Respiration still shallow and costal in type.
    Alæ nasi working slightly.
    Abdominal wall very rigid, tender, and often retracted or flat.
    Tender pelvic peritoneum.
    Diminution of liver-dullness.
    Movable dullness in flanks (sometimes).
    Great pain on movement of the body.

Stage of frank peritonitis with toxic shock :
    Vomiting more frequent.
    Facies that of late peritonitis.
    Abdomen tender and *distended.*
    Pulse rapid and small.
    Temperature either slightly febrile or subnormal.
    Abdominal wall usually not quite so rigid.
    Respiration laboured and rapid.

1. *Stage of primary shock.*—The initial symptoms are those due to the pain and shock consequent on

the flooding of the peritoneal cavity with the gastric contents. The sudden great stimulation of the innumerable nerve-terminations by the irritating fluid escaping from the ruptured viscus causes reflex depression of the vital functions. This may be so severe that the patient may feel faint or fall down in a syncopal attack. The pulse temporarily is small and feeble, the face livid, the extremities cold, and the thermometer will only register about 95° F. The face shows pain and anxiety, and the patient may cry out in his agony.

The pain is sudden in onset. The patient may be feeling well one moment, the next he is writhing in agony and crying out for someone to relieve him. The site of the initial pain is generally epigastric, but quickly it extends downwards, and in a short time is felt all over the abdomen. The pain may even be greater in the hypogastrium, since the escaped fluid collects in the pelvis. This stage may last for but a few minutes or persist for an hour or two. Its length depends to a certain extent upon the size of the perforation and the degree to which the general peritoneal cavity is flooded. In cases where the perforation is very small and soon sealed up by fibrinous exudate the symptoms of onset are correspondingly less severe. In some instances of this kind the shock is almost absent and the pulse may be regular and full when seen shortly after the perforation.

2. *Stage of reaction.*—The intensity of the initial shock subsides, and the patient then looks better and feels more comfortable. The circulatory system recovers to such an extent that the limbs may become warmer, the face normal in colour, and the pulse

normal in frequency and strength, whilst the thermometer may show no indication either of sub-
normality or fever. The improvement in symptoms
does not imply any stoppage of the pathological
process, though the casual observer might easily
think that real improvement were taking place.
Upon the proper appreciation by the practitioner of
this dangerous latent period depends the patient's
chance of recovery from the disease. It is in this
stage that the inexperienced house-surgeon thinks
he has made a mistake in summoning the surgeon
so urgently, and almost apologizes for having
brought him up needlessly. In this stage I have
known a capable observer deluded into postponing
the summons to the surgeon since the patient was
sleeping peacefully. But it is at this period that
the favourable opportunity for operation passes,
nor should there be any difficulty in diagnosis if
careful examination be made.

No certain guide is to be obtained from the pulse
and temperature, for they are frequently normal,
nor is the patient's own opinion of his condition
always to be trusted, for he often expresses himself
as feeling much better, and he may even begin to
think lightly of his condition. But his attitude
and his acts will always belie his words. Relief
will be sought by the drawing up of the legs, and
if he be asked to turn over in bed the attempt is
made cautiously and with evident dread of increasing the pain. If no morphine has been administered
there will still be complaint of generalized abdominal
pain, though the intensity will not be so great as at
first. There are in addition five observations, some
or all of which give valuable indication of the

serious intra-abdominal mischief. **The abdominal wall is rigid and tender, respiration shallow and of costal type, the pelvic peritoneum is tender, and there may be free fluid and free gas in the peritoneal cavity.**

The rigidity of the abdominal wall is a constant feature. The muscles are flat and board-like, and

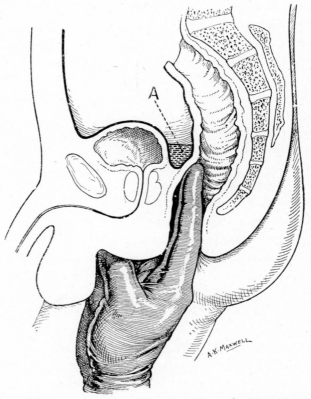

Fig. 15.—Drawing to illustrate how the pelvic peritoneum may be palpated. (*A*) indicates where inflammatory fluid usually collects.

even firm pressure cannot make them give way. It takes a fairly deep anæsthesia to cause them to relax. Pressure on any part of the abdominal wall causes pain, and may evoke retching. Tenderness is often greater in the right iliac fossa in the case of a ruptured duodenal or pyloric ulcer. The rigid muscles do not move on respiration, and the movement of the diaphragm is also considerably inhibited so that

Breathing is shallow and of the costal type.

The *tenderness of the pelvic peritoneum* is a most important sign. This can be determined by a rectal or, in the female, by a vaginal examination. Within a very short time of a perforation the pelvis fills with escaped contents and inflammatory exudate, and, though no lump can be felt, pressure against the pelvic peritoneal pouch through the rectal wall by the inserted finger produces pain which makes the patient wince. Remember, however, that the tenderness of the pelvic peritoneum is not always present if the case is examined within an hour or two of perforation and if the opening be a small one.

Movable dullness in the flanks due to free fluid in the peritoneal cavity should usually be determinable, but the shifting of the patient necessary to elicit the sign is not always advisable. In doubtful cases it may be of value.

The diminution or absence of liver-dullness is the sign produced by free gas in the peritoneal cavity. It is often easily demonstrated, but is frequently ambiguous. Percussion over the front of the liver may produce a resonant note even when no free gas is present in the peritoneal cavity, for it may result from distended intestine which is sometimes pushed up in cases of intestinal obstruction or peritonitis from any cause. If there be no abdominal distension, however, diminution of the liver-dullness anteriorly is significant. It is always of significance to obtain resonance on percussion over the liver in the mid-axillary line. *If in any acute abdominal case distinct resonance be obtained over the liver in the mid-axillary line about two or more inches above the costal border, one is certainly dealing with a perforation of a gastric or duodenal ulcer.* It is only in the minority of cases that the sign is positive.

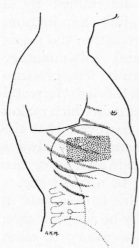

FIG. 16.—Diagram to indicate area of hepatic resonance which is diagnostic of perforation of a gastric, duodenal, or intestinal ulcer.

In doubtful cases, when X-rays are available, it is possible to get great help from a simple radiograph of the diaphragmatic region. By this means small quantities of free gas between the liver and diaphragm may be observed. (See accompanying X-ray, p. 105.)

An additional symptom which may be helpful is the occurrence of pain on the top of the shoulder, either in the supra-spinous fossa, over the acromion, or over the clavicle, i.e. in the region of distribution of the cutaneous branches of the fourth cervical nerve. This symptom, if present, has to be considered carefully with the other indications, for diaphragmatic pleurisy causes similar pain ; but if the pain be felt in both shoulders *from the onset of the attack* it is suggestive of a perforation of the anterior wall of the stomach causing irritation of the median portion of the diaphragm. In the case of a perforation of a pyloric or duodenal ulcer the shoulder pain is usually felt in the right supra-spinous fossa.

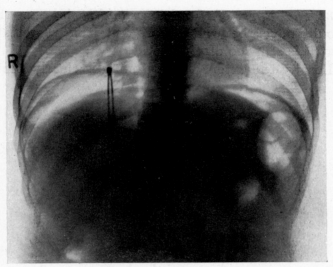

FIG. 17.—X-ray photograph showing free gas between the diaphragm and the upper surface of the liver in a case of perforated duodenal ulcer.

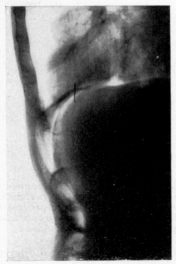

FIG. 18.—X-ray photograph
showing free gas between the
liver and the lateral part of
diaphragm in a case of perforated duodenal ulcer.

3. *The stage of frank peritonitis* is one that should never be waited for, and it is regrettable that it is still too often seen.

Locally the extensive peritonitis is clearly shown

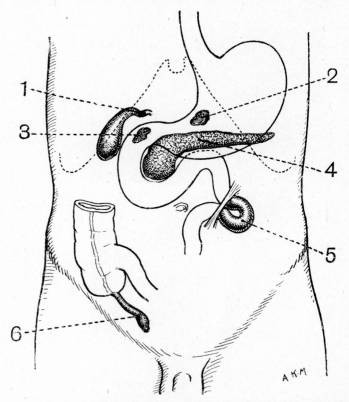

FIG. 19.—Diagram to illustrate the more common abdominal causes of acute collapse: (1) biliary colic; (2) perforated gastric ulcer; (3) perforated duodenal ulcer; (4) acute pancreatitis; (5) acute intestinal obstruction; (6) acute perforative appendicitis. (In the female ruptured ectopic gestation should be added.)

by increasing *distension of the abdomen.* Distension of the abdomen is not a sign of a perforated ulcer—it is an indication that peritonitis is advanced, and that the condition has been allowed to proceed so far that the chance of recovery is slight. Yet I have known delay in sending up a case to hospital, because the one who suspected perforation thought that diagnosis could hardly be sustained in the absence of distension.

The other effects of extensive peritonitis are increasing and persistent vomiting, gradual increase in rate and depreciation in force and volume of the pulse, and the consequent decrease in temperature of the extremities and body generally. The abdomen remains tender, but in late peritonitis the rigidity frequently lessens, owing to the toxic effects on the neuro-muscular system. Finally, as a result of the vomiting and depressed circulation, the face becomes pinched and anxious, the cheeks hollow and the eyes dim and beringed with dark circles, the so-called facies Hippocratica, which is not so much a sign of peritonitis as the mask of death following peritonitis.

Diagnosis and differential diagnosis.—During the initial stage of shock it is nearly always possible to say that there is a condition needing surgical intervention, though the exact nature of the catastrophe may be slightly doubtful. Great help is sometimes obtained from a previous history of chronic indigestion or of duodenal pain, coming on about two hours after food. Quite a number of patients, however, give but a recent history of pain after food. This is more common in the case of young people in whom acute pyloric ulcers appear to be not uncommon; but I have had to deal with a perforated duodenal ulcer in a man of seventy-six who had never previously had any symptoms of indigestion.

If, in one who has been subject to chronic indigestion, sudden collapse and very severe abdominal pain suddenly supervene, and if at the same time the abdominal wall becomes generally rigid, one is justified in suspecting a perforation of an ulcer. If in addition the pelvic peritoneum be tender, and there be resonance over the lateral aspect of the liver, diagnosis is certain.

In the stage of reaction the general symptoms temporarily improve, but *all the local signs remain and become still more definite* so that the careful observer should not be misled. In the third stage, there is no difficulty in diagnosing that some serious catastrophe within the abdomen has occurred.

Differential diagnosis.—There are three conditions sometimes giving rise to symptoms similar to those of perforated ulcer, which either do not call for operation or in which operative interference is positively contra-indicated. They are :

> SEVERE COLIC (either biliary or renal),
> GASTRIC CRISES OF TABES DORSALIS.
> SOME CASES OF PLEURO-PNEUMONIA.

There are five other conditions which always call for operative treatment and which are sometimes difficult to distinguish from a perforated gastric or duodenal ulcer. They are :

> ACUTE PANCREATITIS,
> ACUTE PERFORATIVE APPENDICITIS,
> RUPTURED ECTOPIC GESTATION (IN WOMEN),
> ACUTE INTESTINAL OBSTRUCTION,
> GENERAL OR DIFFUSE PERITONITIS FROM
>   OTHER CAUSES.

Biliary and renal colic may cause severe collapse and terrible abdominal pain. The extent of the collapse is not a differential point, since in biliary colic the patient may sometimes appear *in extremis*, but diagnosis is usually clear on a consideration of the previous history and condition of the abdominal wall, liver-dullness, and pelvic peritoneum. A clear account given of prior attacks of pain and jaundice, or hæmaturia and the passing of gravel or a small stone, would serve to indicate the probability of a stone trying to pass down the biliary ducts or ureter respectively.

The radiation of the pain of biliary colic to the subscapular region, and that of renal colic to the testicle, are sufficiently diagnostic. In stone-colic the abdominal wall is not usually rigid, and the sufferer may throw himself about or writhe in agony while attempting to gain a more easy position. After perforation of an ulcer the general abdominal rigidity and increase of pain on movement forbid and prevent movement, though occasional exceptions occur. Finally the pelvic peritoneum is not tender nor is there any diminution of liver-dullness in biliary or renal colic. If jaundice or hæmaturia be observed, diagnosis will not be in doubt. Renal colic is nearly always strictly limited to one side.

The *gastric crises* of tabes dorsalis may give rise to difficulty in diagnosis, for the intensity of the abdominal pain and the severity of the vomiting may cause extreme collapse. It should be a rule always to test the knee-jerks and the pupillary reactions in every acute abdominal case, for in tabes one or other of these is nearly always abnormal. The patient, moreover, may give a history of pre-

vious similar attacks, and on examination in a
tabetic crisis there will be no rigidity of the abdominal muscles, nor should there be tenderness on
examination per rectum, nor resonance over the
lateral aspect of the liver. It is to be remembered
that a patient may have a perforated ulcer whilst
the subject of tabes, but in such a case some of
the last-mentioned signs will be present. *Persisting
rigidity of the abdominal wall is never due to tabes*,
and tragic misdiagnosis may occur if this point is
not remembered.

Right-sided or bilateral pleuro-pneumonia.—An
acute case of double or right-sided pleuro-pneumonia will sometimes cause considerable abdominal
rigidity, and great epigastric pain, but in such there
are usually sufficient signs in the lung to point to
the true cause of the condition. The alæ nasi will
be working and the respiration-rate will be greater
than one would expect with an early peritonitis
without distension. With pleuro-pneumonia there
is usually fever and a raised pulse-rate. Once more
rectal examination and percussion over the lateral
aspect of the liver are of importance in diagnosis.

The other five conditions are all serious states
which themselves imperatively call for an opening
of the abdomen, so that, though important, it is not
of such critical necessity to make a certain diagnosis
before operating.

Acute pancreatitis simulates visceral perforation
very closely, and before the abdomen is opened is
generally mistaken either for that condition or for
intestinal obstruction. In pancreatitis the pain is
even more agonizing, but the abdominal rigidity is
not so generalized nor so constant. Cyanosis and

slight jaundice are more often seen in pancreatitis, which usually occurs in fat subjects. The diagnosis is further considered in the next section (p. 119).

Acute appendicitis should easily be distinguished by consideration of the history, the order of the symptoms, and the local signs. It is infrequent for inflammation of the appendix to cause such acutely severe symptoms as those ushering in a gastric perforation, but in the stage of reaction a perforated ulcer may be, and often is, misdiagnosed as appendicitis. Especially is this the case with a leaking duodenal ulcer, for the escaped contents may trickle down chiefly on the right side of the abdomen and cause pain particularly in the right iliac fossa. This simulates appendicitis closely, for the sequence —epigastric pain, nausea and vomiting, right iliac pain and fever—may be produced just as in inflammation of the appendix. The intensity of the initial collapse may serve to distinguish, and the persistence of tenderness over the duodenal area should help to determine the condition. In appendicitis the abdominal rigidity is seldom so extensive as in perforated ulcer, and the liver-dullness is normal, though in both cases there may be rectal tenderness. In many cases of perforated duodenal ulcer, the patient may complain of pain on the top of the right shoulder or over the right supra-spinous fossa ; very rarely is shoulder-pain felt in appendicitis, and when felt (due to irritative fluid reaching the diaphragm) the pain would be more likely felt over the acromion or clavicular region. In both cases operation is indicated.

Intestinal obstruction should not give rise to difficulty save in those cases which come late for

diagnosis. Acute strangulation of a coil of small
bowel is the most likely type to cause difficulty.
In both conditions the onset may be with acute
symptoms of collapse, pain, and vomiting and in
both there may be evidence of free fluid in the abdomen, but in obstruction the abdominal wall
is usually flaccid and quite unlike the rigid board-
like condition in perforated ulcer. In acute
obstruction vomiting is almost from the first a
distinctive feature, and the character of the vomit
gradually changes until it is fæculent.

In the late stages of both conditions it may be
difficult to distinguish between them, for peritonitis
is often a complication of late intestinal obstruction,
and the board-like rigidity accompanying a perforated ulcer tends to diminish somewhat as the
distension increases, and as the absorption of
toxins diminishes the neuro-muscular reflex activity. In such cases the history, and possibly the
character of the vomit, may serve to differentiate.

Rupture of an ectopic gestation, leading to severe
intra-peritoneal hæmorrhage, may cause syncope
and collapse, vomiting and severe abdominal pain.
A history of menstrual irregularity may be obtained,
but one must not rely on that for diagnosis. The
main points in diagnosis are the blanching of the lips,
tongue, nails, and sclerotics and the absence of true
abdominal rigidity, though the abdomen is generally
tender and tumid, especially in the lower part. In
both cases there will be some tenderness on digital
rectal or vaginal examination. No definite pelvic
swelling can be made out in most cases of recent
rupture of an ectopic gestation. Free fluid in the
abdomen may be detectable in both conditions,

and resonance over the *front* of the liver may be obtainable sometimes with a ruptured ectopic gestation (due to intestine pushed up by clots of blood), but resonance over the lateral aspect of the liver is only obtained with a perforated ulcer.

Pain over the clavicles or in the supra-spinous fossa is sometimes a complaint in cases of ruptured extra-uterine gestation as with perforated ulcer. This is due to diaphragmatic irritation by the clotted blood in the upper abdomen.

Other forms of peritonitis can only be distinguished from that due to a perforated ulcer by considering the history of onset, and by determining the presence or absence of gas on the lateral aspect of the liver. It may be impossible to differentiate from the results of perforation of some other part of the gut. Peritonitis due to rupture of the gall-bladder may be accompanied by an icteric tinge in the conjunctivæ.

(B) RUPTURE OF AN ULCER WITH FORMATION OF LOCALIZED SUBPHRENIC ABSCESS

When from one reason or another—previous adhesions, slow leakage allowing time for deposit of fibrin—the escaping gastric contents do not flood the peritoneal cavity, the symptoms are correspondingly modified. The pain may be very great, but the initial collapse is not so prostrating, and the abdominal signs will soon localize themselves to the upper segment of the abdomen and lead to the development of a subphrenic abscess containing gas. If such an abscess develops anteriorly, the local signs of intra-peritoneal suppuration are very evident, but when the mischief is high up under the diaphragm the signs and symptoms take longer to develop. Irregular temperature, rigors, leucocytosis, and dullness at the base of the lung consequent on pleural effusion or basal congestion, will lead the observer to diagnose a collection of pus under the diaphragm. A full description of subphrenic abscess does not come within the scope of this book.

It must be remembered that occasionally an ulcer may perforate and allow a small leak, but the perforation may soon be sealed by a fibrin-deposit. Such cases give rise to pain, rigidity and tenderness in the right hypochondrium closely simulating the symptoms of acute cholecystitis, and the condition may clear up without the formation of abscess.

ACUTE PANCREATITIS

Acute pancreatitis accounts for less than 1 per cent. of the cases of acute abdominal disease and must therefore be regarded as a comparatively rare disease. It must be exceptional for any one surgeon to see more than two or three dozen cases in the course of his career, so that dogmatic views based on personal experience alone must be (as in this case they are) supplemented and corrected by careful study of the experience of others.

It has been stated that the common failure to diagnose acute pancreatitis correctly is due to neglect to consider its possibility in the individual case, but even when the condition is thoroughly considered and discussed a mistaken diagnosis frequently results. Probably less than half the cases are correctly diagnosed before operation. A special consideration of the symptoms is therefore all the more necessary.

To understand and remember the symptoms one should recollect the anatomy of the pancreas and the pathology of the disease. The gland lies in the retro-peritoneal tissues in close relationship with the cœliac plexus and the semilunar ganglia. The head is surrounded by and slightly overlaps the curve of the duodenum ; the body lies in front of the first lumbar vertebra, whilst the tail reaches the left loin and lies against the spleen. There are still many points in the pathology of pancreatitis which are not settled ; but there is a preponderance of evidence to show that the acute forms of inflammation are almost always due to infection which leads to severe and widespread hæmorrhage into the gland, with subsequent disorganization of its substance and liberation and activation of its ferments. If the patient lives long enough a part or the whole of the pancreas may become gangrenous.

Acute pancreatitis seldom occurs before the age of forty, and is more common in stout people ; it may or may not be associated with gall-stones, and the stopping up of the ampulla of Vater by a stone which may divert the bile along the pancreatic duct is an uncommon accompaniment of the disease.

The symptoms of acute pancreatitis are rather variable—a fact which explains the conflicting accounts of the disease published by individual observers. The one or two pathognomonic symptoms are rarely present, and the more constant features must be carefully considered together before a diagnosis can be determined. It is better to group the manifestations according to their cause.

I. Symptoms due to **inflammatory tension of the gland.**

1. **Pain.**—Though there may have been slight attacks of pain prior to the main attack, the acute onset is usually dramatically sudden, and fainting may occur. The pain is excruciating and the patient will cry out in agony. It is felt in the epigastric zone and *in one or both loins*. The position of the gland accounts for the loin-pain, and the neighbourhood of the cœliac plexus explains its severity. Sometimes pain is felt in the left scapular region and occasionally in the left supra-spinous fossa (phrenic pain). Later on the intensity of the pain diminishes, but it may be felt over the whole abdomen or perhaps more *in the right iliac fossa*.

2. **Shock.**—Profound shock usually accompanies the pain. The cold extremities, sweating skin, weak pulse, and subnormal temperature sufficiently witness to the severity of the shock. The thermometer may register as low as 95° F. The pulse is usually rapid and weak, but I have known it slow and full even in the early stage of an attack, when the other symptoms of shock were very evident.

3. **Reflex vomiting** or **retching** nearly always occurs. Sometimes the retching is incessant, but as a rule very little material is brought up. The vomiting is more persistent than with a perforated ulcer. Occasionally no nausea is felt. In true reflex vomiting the vomit is never fæculent.

4. **Local epigastric tenderness** is a constant finding.

5. **Epigastric rigidity** is by no means constant. It is true that soon after the onset there may be board-like rigidity of the epigastric muscles, *but* when the patient is examined there is *often a lax abdominal wall*. Of sixteen cases recorded by

Waring and Griffith [1] thirteen had a soft abdominal wall. This point should be emphasized, since extreme muscular rigidity was at one time thought to be characteristic.

II. Symptoms due to **swelling of the pancreas.**

6. **Epigastric tumour.**—Sometimes the pancreas may be palpable as a transversely placed tumour in the epigastrium. The fact that the patients are usually very stout and the occasional presence of rigidity often make the detection of the tumour difficult.

7. **Jaundice.**—Slight jaundice is found in about half the cases. Since frequently, if not usually, there are no obstructing gall-stones, the most reasonable explanation for the jaundice is that the common duct is compressed by the swollen head of the pancreas. The common duct is normally surrounded by the head of the gland in two out of three cases.

8. **Obstructive vomiting.** — True obstructive vomiting of great amounts of fæculent or bilious material is very rare, but I have personal knowledge of one such case. At the operation the swollen pancreatic head was definitely obstructing the duodenum. This type of vomit must be distinguished from the more common reflex vomiting mentioned above.

III. Symptoms due to **extravasation of blood.**

9. **Ecchymosis of one or both loins** is an occasional symptom (Grey-Turner's sign). The extravasated blood finds its way along the retro-peritoneal tissue planes and becomes evident as a greenish-yellow or purplish stain in the loin external

[1] See *British Journal of Surgery*, vol. xi, p. 476. We wish to express our indebtedness to this article, which we consider one of the most valuable yet written on the subject.

to the erector spinæ muscle-mass. This symptom can only appear after two or three days from the onset of the disease. When present it is absolutely pathognomonic.

IV. Symptoms due to **deranged gland function.**

10. **Glycosuria** is occasionally found, and in any case of acute abdominal pain should raise the question of pancreatic disease.

11. **Increase in the urinary diastase.**—The liberation of the pancreatic ferments leads to an increase in the amount of diastase in the urine. Normally the urine contains about 10 to 20 units of diastase, but in acute pancreatitis this may be increased to 100 or 200 units. Facilities for this test are, however, not always handy, and it is not always reliable.

V. **Other symptoms.**

12. **Cyanosis.**—This symptom has been noted in a considerable number of cases. It is best observed in the face and extremities, but has sometimes been present in the skin of the abdomen.

13. Dyspnœa is occasionally noticeable. It is reasonable to suppose that a partial inhibition of the diaphragmatic movements, owing to the contiguous inflammation, may account at any rate in part for the cyanosis and dyspnœa.

14. Loewi's test or adrenaline mydriasis is sometimes positive. A drop or two of a 1 in 1,000 adrenaline hydrochloride solution is dropped into one conjunctival sac and the procedure repeated in five minutes. Within half an hour the pupil on the tested side only should dilate if the test is positive. The test indicates disturbance of the suprarenals by contiguous disease, and is found

occasionally in acute pancreatitis, but it has been known to be positive in cases of hyperthyroidism.

It should be remembered that in the later stages of acute pancreatitis a more general abdominal condition results ; blood-stained fluid collects in the peritoneal cavity, distension supervenes, and there may be irregular fever. It is very difficult to diagnose such cases without a very accurate previous history of the case.

Diagnosis.—Acute pancreatitis is most commonly mistaken for a *perforated gastric or duodenal ulcer*. The less acute cases may be misdiagnosed *appendicitis*, whilst those cases with distension may easily be regarded as examples of *intestinal obstruction*. *Acute cholecystitis* and *biliary colic* may also simulate the symptoms of pancreatitis.

With a perforated ulcer general abdominal rigidity is constant in the early stages after perforation, whilst in pancreatitis the abdomen may be softer, and any rigidity is usually limited to the epigastric zone. In his original paper, Fitz very accurately wrote that the symptoms of acute pancreatitis were those of an *epigastric* peritonitis. In a case of perforated ulcer the symptoms are usually more widespread. Pain on top of the shoulder is frequently felt when an ulcer perforates ; with pancreatitis such pain is rare, and when present is felt on top of the left shoulder. Bilateral lumbar pain, cyanosis, and slight jaundice would be in favour of pancreatitis, whilst absence of liver-dullness in the axillary line would definitely indicate perforated ulcer. Glycosuria, a positive Loewi test, or (when the test can be made) a great increase in the diastase content of the urine, would point to pancreatitis.

Appendicitis is generally distinguishable if careful attention be paid to the history of onset and the order of symptoms. The vomiting and pain are both less severe in appendicitis, and there may be definite local symptoms in the right iliac fossa. With acute cholecystitis and biliary colic tenderness is felt more in the right hypochondrium, and there may be a definite history of previous attacks, whilst hyperæsthesia to pin-stroke in the superficial distribution of the 8th or 9th thoracic nerves may point to gall-bladder trouble. The tests of glandular derangement may help to determine, but it must be remembered that cholecystitis and pancreatitis may co-exist.

When distension has supervened it is difficult to distinguish from the late stages of peritonitis and intestinal obstruction unless positive tests of deranged gland-function and a very clear history point to the correct diagnosis.

With every care in investigation acute pancreatitis is frequently only diagnosed with certainty when the abdomen is opened and blood-stained fluid and areas of fat-necrosis are seen.

CHAPTER VII

ACUTE INTESTINAL OBSTRUCTION

Acute obstruction of the intestine in the form of strangulated hernia was one of the first of the abdominal emergencies to be referred to the surgeon for treatment, whilst obstruction accompanied by similar symptoms, but due to internal causes which were not so obvious as an external hernial swelling, was amongst the latest of the urgent abdominal cases to be given up by the physician to the surgeon. Medical treatment was, a generation ago, recommended to be tried as a first resort, and only when a course of treatment by aperients and enemata failed to relieve was the operating colleague called in to see the patient. If there be any condition in which early diagnosis and operative treatment, and avoidance of attempts at purgation, are necessary, it is intestinal obstruction. For a patient to be allowed to continue in violent pain, and to vomit repeatedly whilst the abdomen gradually becomes distended, is unfair not only to the patient but also to the surgeon who may have to operate in conditions made so much worse by delay.

The pathology and causation of acute intestinal obstruction are far too big questions to discuss fully in a small book. We are here concerned only with the common causes and the main types of cases

121

which come for diagnosis. It is not always essential in diagnosis to know the exact cause of the obstruction, though every effort should be made to ascertain it as accurately as possible. It is useful to have a knowledge of the proportion of cases due to the main pathological causes of obstruction. In a consecutive series of 301 cases of intestinal obstruction at St. Mary's Hospital, 177 were due to strangulated hernia and 124 to all other causes combined. It is a mistake to treat strangulated external hernia in a different category from obstruction in which no external cause is to be found. Strangulated hernia is the most common form of intestinal obstruction, and is responsible for many more deaths than any other single cause of that condition (see Chapter I). Apart from strangulated external hernia there are only three *common* forms of intestinal obstruction—intussusception, carcinoma of the large bowel, and obstruction by adhesions or bands. Volvulus, gall-stone obstruction, fibrous and tuberculous stricture of the gut and all the rarer causes are responsible for only about 15 per cent. of the cases. The very rough generalization may be made that in infancy acute obstructive symptoms are usually due to intussusception ; in childhood, adolescence, and early middle age to bands and adhesions ; and in later life to cancerous stricture of the large bowel. Adhesions or bands attached to the region around a formerly inflamed appendix are responsible for many cases, whilst a Meckel's diverticulum is in younger life responsible for some band-obstructions.

When the bowel is obstructed so that nothing can

pass the obstruction the course of the disease is inevitably towards a fatal issue unless the obstruction be relieved either by :

(*a*) The spontaneous rectification of the condition —which is almost unknown save in a few cases of reduction of an obstructed hernia, and the occasional cure of an intussusception by the sloughing of the invaginated part ;

(*b*) Formation of an external fæcal fistula ; or,

(*c*) Operative interference.

The third method is in all cases desirable. Until comparatively recently the mortality after operation in cases of intestinal obstruction (excluding strangulated external herniæ) was well over 50 per cent., and even now it is more than it should be because the patients are not operated upon early enough. The main desideratum is to diagnose the cases early. There are few cases of intestinal obstruction which could not be remedied or alleviated if brought to the surgeon within twelve hours of the onset of symptoms.

Intestinal obstruction may exist in a chronic or subacute form for a considerable period before a really acute attack ensues. In the chronic form the symptoms are similar in kind but different in degree from those resulting from an acute attack. Chronic obstruction sooner or later terminates in an acute attack.

The symptoms of acute intestinal obstruction differ greatly according to the site of obstruction. The higher up in the gut is the stoppage, the more severe are the symptoms. It is usually possible to say approximately what part of the gut is obstructed, and cases may be divided roughly into three classes

—those due to obstruction of (1) upper small-gut,
(2) lower small-gut, (3) large bowel, respectively.

General symptoms of acute intestinal obstruction :

Pain.
Shock.
Vomiting.
Constipation (inability to pass fæces or flatus).
Distension.
Tenderness of abdomen.
Visible peristalsis.

Pain is usually very severe from the onset. It is
referred to the epigastric and umbilical regions, or
even sometimes to the hypogastrium, and frequently
comes on in bouts or spasms, though if a considerable segment of mesentery is implicated the pain
may be continuous. The spasmodic pain is due
to the peristalsis of the intestine trying to overcome
the obstruction. This can easily be demonstrated
during the examination of an intussusception, when
the soft tumour may be felt to harden just before
the screaming of the infant. The initial pain is
similar to that caused by any severe stimulation of
the abdominal sympathetic, and is often accompanied by those symptoms consequent on such
stimulation and comprised under the term " shock."

Primary shock or collapse.—In severe cases the
pulse may be weak, the skin cold and sweating, the
temperature subnormal, and the pupils dilated, but
as a rule the symptoms are not so severe as this,
and in most cases of severe primary shock a reaction
follows, and the patient though still in pain appears
and feels a little better.

Vomiting is an almost constant feature, but varies

very greatly in the different forms. The higher up in the intestine the obstruction, the sooner vomiting sets in and the more violent is the regurgitation. In obstruction of the large bowel vomiting may be absent but nausea is constant. In obstructive vomiting, first the stomach contents are expelled, then green bilious material appears, and, if the obstruction be some way down the small intestine, the vomit gradually changes to yellow or greenish brown and becomes fæculent. A fæculent vomit, in the absence of peritonitis, is diagnostic of intestinal obstruction, though it should be regarded as a late symptom of that condition. The nature of the vomit is therefore to be watched very carefully, and the vomited material should never be thrown away till seen by the medical attendant. True fæcal vomit is only seen when a communication exists between the colon and stomach.

Constipation is one of the symptoms of intestinal obstruction, but it is not always evident at first. If the bowel be occluded at any spot, it is clear that no contents can pass the occluded area, but the gut below the stoppage can empty itself, so that for a time the bowels may be opened. So soon as the lower bowel is emptied (either naturally or by enemata) neither flatus nor fæces pass. In doubtful or subacute cases the plan of giving two turpentine enemata with an interval of a few hours (as suggested by Barnard) is good. The first empties the lower bowel, and the second proves or disproves the existence of obstruction. But it is conceivable that both enemata might bring a return of fæcal material and yet obstruction exist. In very acute cases the shock is so great that the gut

may be too paralysed to allow any natural movement of the bowels, though an enema may evacuate
fæcal contents. There are many acute cases in
which constipation should be regarded as a sequel
rather than a symptom, for valuable time may

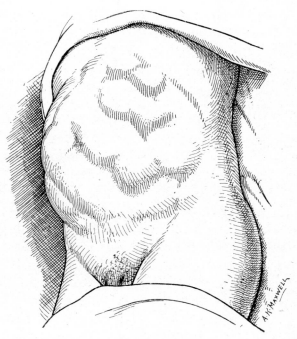

FIG. 20.—Drawing to show ladder pattern of abdominal distension (indicating obstruction of the lower ileum).

be lost in the attempt either to open the bowels
or prove that the obstruction exists. *If the other
symptoms of intestinal obstruction are present it is
unwise to wait twelve or twenty-four hours to demonstrate constipation.* It is advisable to point out
that in acute intussusception there is occasionally
incomplete obstruction, so that some brown or

yellowish fæcal material may come away in addition to the blood and mucus.

Distension is usually late in appearing in the

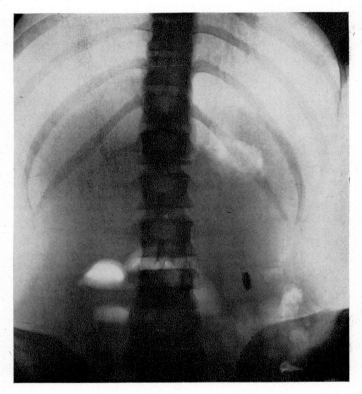

Fig. 21.—Plain X-ray of the abdomen of a lady aged 36 suffering from acute obstruction of the small bowel caused by a band. Spasms af acute abdominal pain had begun a few hours previously, but she had only vomited once. Note the gas held up behind the obstruction which is confirmed by the clearly defined fluid levels. The X-ray indicated the need for immediate operation at which the band was successfully divided.

acute cases, or in those in which the upper part of the small intestine is affected. But always sooner or later it is in evidence. In obstruction of the large bowel and lower end of the small bowel it may be apparent by the time the symptoms become acute enough to call the serious attention of the patient. It is indeed because of the relative slightness of the symptoms—pain and vomiting—that the distension is allowed to proceed so far.

Distension at first may be merely local, owing to the dilatation of the coils of gut immediately above the obstruction. In some cases where ordinary clinical examination does not show any definite distension a radiograph may reveal local distension of the intestine. (Fig. 21.) In obstruction of the end of the ileum a local hypogastric distension may first be observed, and in volvulus of the sigmoid the outline of the affected coil of large bowel may stand out very distinctly. In subacute or partial obstruction of the lower end of the small bowel the distension gradually dilates to a moderate degree coil after coil, so that when the patient comes under observation with acute symptoms the typical ladder-pattern type of distension is seen on looking at the abdomen. (Fig. 20.)

Tenderness of the abdomen is not usually seen till distension appears. Pressure over a distended coil is generally painful. In the later stages of obstruction when peritonitis has ensued there may be general pain all over the abdomen. *Rigidity* of the abdominal wall is unusual save in those cases where there is some local peritonitis round the obstructed area.

Visible peristalsis is not a constant accompaniment of obstruction, but is diagnostic when present, except in some few very thin persons in whom the normal peristaltic movements of the intestines can easily be seen through the abdominal wall.

It is not usually seen in the very acute cases of strangulation, but in subacute obstruction it is more frequently noted and is very valuable in diagnosis. In some instances peristalsis may be accompanied by a gurgling of gas, which may occasionally be heard to pass through a narrowed part of the gut.

Types of obstruction.—The features of an attack of obstruction vary according to (1) the part of gut obstructed, (2) whether the mesentery with the contained blood-vessels is also affected, and (3) the completeness or otherwise of the obstruction.

(1) The symptoms due to obstruction—(*a*) high up in the small intestine ; (*b*) low down in the small intestine ; and (*c*) in the large bowel—can be roughly differentiated.

(*a*) Obstruction high up in the small gut leads to acute symptoms, vomiting comes on very early and is frequent and violent, initial shock and pain are greater, and distension is not an early feature. The vomit is green and bilious. Such symptoms are typically seen when a large gall-stone ulcerates into the duodenum (a rare occurrence). Obstruction of the duodenum by a cicatrized ulcer may sometimes be acute owing to sudden spasm and œdema round the ulcer. In such cases everything taken by mouth is returned, but no fæculent vomit occurs and sometimes peristalsis of the stomach may be seen. Distension is only seen in the epigastric region. With obstruction of the upper jejunum the symptoms are still very acute and the vomiting begins early and is frequently repeated, while distension is not at first a noticeable feature unless there be a strangulation of a large coil of gut. The farther down the jejunum the obstruction the less acute the symptoms.

(*b*) In obstruction of the lower part of the small intestine the symptoms are less severe than those just summarized. Shock and pain may be great,

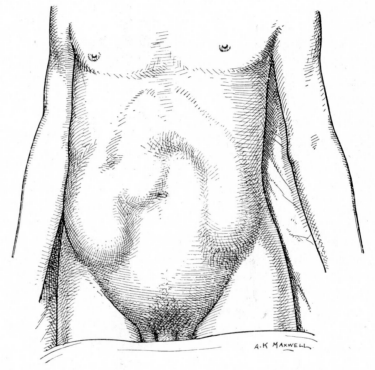

FIG. 22 —Diagram to show appearance of moderate distension of the large gut.

but vomiting is usually a little later in onset ; and some time elapses before fæculent vomit occurs. Distension comes on after a few hours. In subacute cases the ladder pattern of distension is seen, and peristalsis is often visible.

(*c*) In large-bowel obstruction pain is much less

acute, shock is comparatively insignificant (except in some cases of volvulus and intussusception), vomiting is a fairly late and infrequent symptom, whilst distension from the onset of the acute attack is the rule. An exception must be made in the case of intussusception, for in these cases distension is not an early symptom and should not be waited for, since a distended abdomen accompanying an intussusception generally means that the chance of recovery is slight.

(2) When the vessels in the mesentery of a coil of gut are compressed first the veins and later the arteries become occluded, and the gut soon becomes gangrenous. There is local peritonitis round the affected coil. The obstruction of the gut is necessarily complete. This condition is commonly brought about by bands, by external or internal hernia, or by volvulus. The onset of symptoms is usually sudden, accompanied by collapse or severe shock, great pain, and early vomiting. If the gut is completely within the abdomen the local peritonitis will tend to become more general, and by the time the case comes to the surgeon there may therefore be definite abdominal rigidity over the affected part of the abdomen.

(3) The symptoms of obstruction vary greatly with the degree of occlusion of the lumen of the gut. When the obstruction is partial, or if the muscular contractions can to any extent force the contents past the obstructed part, the symptoms are less severe. This may result from a kinking of the gut due to adhesions between the bowel and either a calcified gland, the abdominal wall, or another viscus or tumour. In these cases the onset is

more insidious, the pain is not so severe and may have intervals of intermission, the vomiting may for a day or two be slight in degree, and distension comes on but gradually. Quite commonly such cases do not come to the surgeon until fæculent vomit has appeared. In these cases the abdominal wall is quite flaccid, since peritonitis is absent, for the gut remains intact, and its blood-supply in the mesentery is unimpaired. This type is the variety which may occur after abdominal operations, when a certain amount of pain, vomiting and distension is usually to be expected. There is therefore all the greater need to watch such cases carefully.

In the gradual narrowing of the gut-lumen due to stricture, subacute volvulus, or chronic intussusception, and in cases where only a part of the lumen of the bowel is nipped in a hernial aperture (Richter's hernia), the onset of symptoms is still more gradual, vomiting is less, and the pain is intermittent.

A Richter's hernia of the cæcum (of which one instance has occurred in the author's practice) may be unaccompanied by any obstruction of the bowel and the herniated part of the gut-wall may become gangrenous without giving rise to any acute symptoms.

When omentum only is strangulated there are subacute symptoms of obstruction, pain, vomiting, and some distension, but the vomiting never becomes fæculent, and the obstruction is never complete—for flatus and fæces are brought away by enemata. The general symptoms in omental strangulation are usually slight, but if a large mass becomes gangrenous (e.g. in an umbilical hernia) serious symptoms and even death may result.

Diagnosis of small-gut obstruction.—When a patient is seized with acute abdominal pain, becomes collapsed with feeble pulse, cold extremities, anxious look and sweating skin, and soon begins to vomit first the stomach contents, then bile, then yellowish material which becomes brownish and fæculent-smelling, while the abdomen remains flaccid, flat, and not tender, that patient is suffering from acute obstruction of the small intestine. The diagnosis should be made without waiting for distension to appear, nor—if the above symptoms are present—is there any need to demonstrate constipation. If the symptoms are not so acute there will be additional signs, for there is an inverse proportion between the acuteness of the symptoms and the probability of the presence of signs. When pain and vomiting and shock are slight, distension and visible peristalsis are more likely to be seen and constipation, tested by two turpentine enemata, can usually be demonstrated. Thus it is that when acute supervenes upon chronic obstruction both symptoms and signs are in evidence.

Differential diagnosis of acute obstruction of the small intestine.—Diagnosis must be considered either before distension has developed or after that sign has appeared. In any case, *always examine first all the hernial orifices*.

When no distension is present acute obstruction has to be distinguished from all the other acute abdominal catastrophes. The pain is often characteristic in type, occurring in bouts of acute intensity during which the severity is reflected in the patient's drawn features ; it is usually central in position except in those cases in which a coil is strangled, when the pain will be referred to the site of strangulation. Sometimes borborygmi may be heard passing along the bowel. During the intervals between the bouts the patient's face shows apprehension of the return of the pain. From the acute inflammations—perforated gastric ulcer, pancreatitis, appendicitis with peritonitis, cholecystitis—it is distinguished by the absence of rigidity and by the more frequent vomiting *which tends to become fæculent.* Renal and biliary colic are distinguished by the location and radiation of the pain and the absence of fæculent vomit. Neither stoppage of the bowel contents nor distension follows the colics. In torsion of a viscus (ovarian cyst, testicle) the vomiting does not become fæculent. Gastric crisis is excluded by finding no other sign of tabes. It is usually sufficient to test the knee-jerks and the pupillary reactions.

In many cases in which the diagnosis of obstruction of the small intestine is in question great help may be obtained from a study of a plain X-ray of the abdomen. Normally little or no gas or fluid can be seen in the regions of the abdomen occupied by small-gut. When there is obstruction, however, the contents are dammed back, and a plain skiagram will often show small collections of gas, each lying on top of a minute pool of liquid whose fluid level is characteristic. This aid is particularly helpful in the early stages of obstruction of the upper jejunum when no distension is likely to be present.

When distension is present one must consider the question of uræmia, mesenteric thrombosis or embolism, or the late stage of peritonitis due to any cause.

Uræmia should be diagnosed by careful consideration of the history, by examination of the urine for albumin, and maybe by detecting enlargement of the kidneys. Sometimes in uræmic patients there may be a mere trace of albumin in the urine, but a low specific gravity would make one suspicious, and examination of the heart and determination of the blood-pressure may throw light on the case.

Acute blockage of the mesenteric arteries or veins by an embolus or thrombus may lead to symptoms indistinguishable from those due to internal strangulation. In both cases the vascular disturbance leads rapidly to serious changes in the bowel. With primary mesenteric thrombosis the extent of gut affected is likely to be greater, and distension of the abdomen appears more rapidly. Sometimes a palpable mass is formed by the affected coil or gut. A history of recent endocarditis might point to a possible embolism, whilst hepatic disease or previous thrombotic trouble would sometimes suggest the possibility of mesenteric thrombosis. Though there is no mechanical obstruction in the intestines in a case of vascular occlusion, the affected gut soon becomes paralysed and hæmorrhagic, and the blood which is almost always poured into the bowel lumen as a consequence of the infarction sometimes passes into the gut farther on and can be demonstrated by the administration of an enema (Cokkinis).

Unless promptly dealt with, mesenteric thrombosis is soon followed by peritonitis.

It may be impossible to distinguish between a late

case of intestinal obstruction and late peritonitis, unless the history gives some indication. In late peritonitis there is usually paralytic intestinal obstruction, whilst in the late stages of mechanical obstruction there is frequently peritonitis. In peritonitis, however, the vomit is seldom so definitely fæculent as in late mechanical obstruction.

Obstruction of the small intestine by a gall-stone can sometimes be distinguished by certain features first described by Barnard.

A gall-stone which causes obstruction generally ulcerates into the duodenum, causing the symptoms of very acute obstruction, i.e. severe pain and frequent vomiting of everything taken into the stomach. The vomit may contain blood from the ulcerated opening, and this may lead to an erroneous diagnosis of gastric ulcer. The stone passes on gradually and the symptoms abate considerably, but in a day or two it stops again at the lower end of the ileum (which is the narrowest part of the small intestine) and the symptoms recur. Therefore if one is faced with a case showing symptoms of obstruction of the *upper* small-gut in which these symptoms subside but are followed in a day or two by those suggestive of obstruction of the *lower* small-gut, the cause is likely to be a gall-stone. This is the more likely if there has been a history suggestive of gall-stones or if the patient is a fat woman of middle or advanced age. Occlusion of the small intestine by a gall-stone is the only type of obstruction in which I have seen fæculent vomiting come on very early and persist (with diminishing frequency) without any serious collapse or abdominal distension supervening. What little distension

develops may be concealed by a fat abdominal wall
so that the abdomen may actually appear normal.

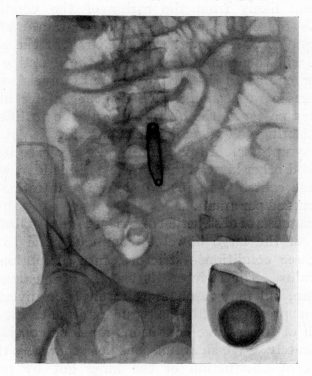

FIG. 23.—Plain X-ray of the abdomen of a lady aged 80
with intestinal obstruction due to a gall-stone which
can be seen in the lower ileum. The inset shows the
radiologically opaque part in relation to the whole
stone. The patient had a past history entirely free
from abdominal symptoms. The illness began with
acute symptoms which eased off but returned 3 days
later. She made a good recovery after removal of
the stone.

The character of the vomit remains fæculent though
there may be longer intervals between the bouts
of pain and vomiting. Considerable distension may
develop towards the end of the case. The above

characters make gall-stone obstruction of the small intestine more easy to diagnose than would be considered likely from the rarity of the condition. Some of these large gall-stones contain material opaque to X-rays, and a plain X-ray of the abdomen will then show the stone in the intestine and guide one as to the best place for the incision. If the radiograph should give evidence of air in the biliary passages, the observer would be justified in considering gall-stone ileus as the probable cause of the symptoms. In one case under my care it also showed other large stones in the gall-bladder, which in due course were passed along the intestine and evacuated per anum.

Diagnosis of obstruction of the large gut.—Obstruction of the large bowel is commonly due to one of three conditions—stricture, intussusception, or volvulus. The stricture is usually of a cancerous nature, but may result more rarely from diverticulitis or pressure of fibrous tissue external to the gut. Each of these three conditions must be considered separately. We shall not consider separately those cases of obstruction of the large gut by pelvic tumours, since the primary condition is usually evident.

CHAPTER VIII

INTUSSUSCEPTION

INTUSSUSCEPTION or invagination of the intestine is the most common abdominal emergency in children under two years. It is much less common in later childhood and adult life, only 30 per cent. of cases occurring after the second year of life. The catastrophe is all the more unexpected in that it usually attacks the most healthy-looking and well-nourished babies. The condition consists in the invagination of one portion of intestine into the portion next to it. Commonly, if not invariably, the invaginated part (intussusceptum) enters the part below (intussuscipiens). Clearly the most anatomically favourable part for such an occurrence is in the ileo-cæcal region, where the narrow ileum can readily enter the lax cæcum, and in actual clinical experience this is the most common place for the condition to start (Fig. 24). There are three varieties of intussusception—enteric, entero-colic, and colic. Enteric, where the small intestine alone is involved, is uncommon ; colic, in which the colon alone is affected, is less rare but not very common ; entero-colic is the most common variety. The entero-colic type is subdivided into ileo-cæcal, in which the apex of the invaginated part is the ileo-cæcal valve, and ileo-colic, in which a part of the gut near the end of the ileum forms the advancing apex.

In the case of the most common form—the entero-colic—as the end of the ileum is invaginated into the colon a portion of the mesentery goes with it

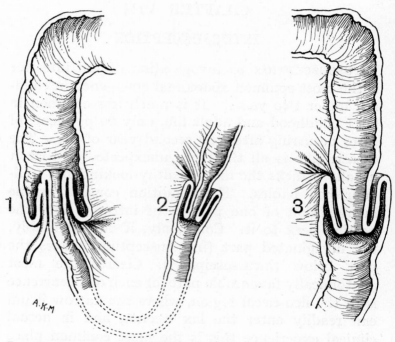

FIG. 24.—Types of intussusception : (1) ileo-cæcal; (2) enteric (which is termed "ileo-colic" if it progress beyond the ileo-cæcal valve); (3) colic.

and constriction, and later strangulation, of the vessels occur, causing œdema of the gut-wall with intestinal hæmorrhage and finally gangrene. The irritation caused by the intruded gut leads to an excessive secretion of mucus. The part of the gut which first becomes invaginated remains at the apex of the advancing portion, and it progresses at the expense of the ensheathing layer (intussuscipiens). The apex is sometimes extruded at the anus. If left untreated intussusception ends in one of two ways. Most commonly the intestinal lumen is gradually occluded, and acute intestinal obstruction and death from toxæmia or peritonitis result ; or more rarely the invaginated part becomes completely gangrenous, and passes per anum as a large slough In pre-operative days many such cases were recorded, but, since it was a comparative rarity for infants to recover from the condition, such a fortunate event as a natural cure by gangrene of the intussuscepted part was usually recorded.

The cause of intussusception appears to be the presence in the gut of something which provokes excessive peristalsis. It commonly occurs in infants at the weaning-time, when there are likely to be occasional portions of undigestible solid food taken by the well-nourished baby. In later life tumours of the gut-wall are commonly the cause of the condition.

The symptoms of intussusception are usually characteristic. They comprise a few or many of the following according to the stage at which the case is seen.

(1) Abdominal pain.
(2) Shock.
(3) Passage of blood and mucus per anum.
(4) Vomiting.
(5) An abdominal swelling.
(6) Visible peristalsis.
(7) Constipation.
(8) Absence of cæcum from the right iliac fossa.

(9) Tenesmus.

(10) Distension of abdomen.

(11) Appearance of apex of intussusception at anus.

(12) Peritonitis.

(1) The onset is usually with a *fit of screaming*—the infant's method of indicating pain. The legs are drawn up during the screaming attacks. The pain is very severe, but is not continuous, and corresponds to the violent peristaltic contraction of the gut. Between the bouts of pain the child may lie quiet, but often has an apprehensive look. Less often the child does not scream or show any sign of abdominal pain other than pallor and drawing up of the legs or restlessly rolling over on the bed.

(2) The severity of the pain is shown by the *symptoms of shock* which accompany it. The extreme facial pallor, the dilated pupils, and anxious appearance of the child are sufficiently demonstrative.

(3) At a period varying according to the site of the invagination—later if it starts in the ileum, earlier if in the transverse colon—*blood and mucus are passed per anum.* This usually occurs within a few hours. The blood is often quite slight in amount, and it is seldom copious. Slimy mucus is mixed with the blood, and not infrequently some brown or yellow fæcal material may also be passed. Cases do occur, however, in which no blood is passed per anum before the child comes under observation sometimes up to as long as 24 or 48 hours after onset of the pain. The practitioner must be prepared to diagnose intussusception before blood has been passed per anum.

(4) *Vomiting* generally occurs, but it is not severe

at first. It is never a serious feature until the late stages when obstruction has ensued or peritonitis developed. The contents of the stomach are returned, any liquid taken is not retained by

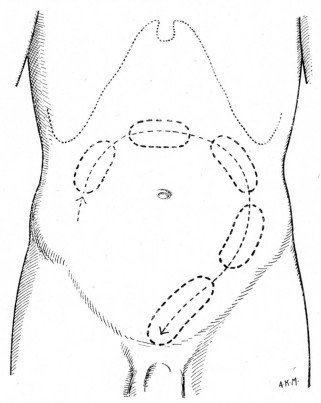

Fig. 25.—Diagram to show possible positions of abdominal tumour in cases of intussusception.

the viscus, and later there may be bilious vomit, but fæculent vomit is rare.

(5) By the time blood appears per anum *a tumour* will be present in the abdomen. It is caused by the invaginated gut, and is felt either in the

right loin, right hypochondrium, epigastrium, left hypochondrium, left lumbar region or left iliac region, according to the advance made by the intussusception through the colon. The tumour is

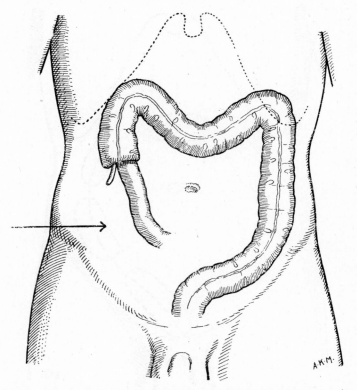

FIG. 26.—Diagram to show how the cæcum is absent from the right iliac fossa in intussusception. (This is a valuable diagnostic point in distinguishing from colitis.)

oval in shape, and has often been compared—quite aptly—to a sausage. Sometimes the swelling becomes harder, the change corresponding to the muscular peristaltic contraction. Frequently it is easy to feel the swelling, but in many cases an anæsthetic is necessary to relax the abdominal wall, and even when the child is anæsthetized it may be difficult to identify an intussusception which lies under cover of the liver. *The hiding of the intussusception by the overhanging liver is responsible for many failures to detect the tumour.*

(6) *Peristalsis* may sometimes be seen through the abdominal wall, and the simultaneous hardening of the tumour has been referred to above.

(7) In the common entero-colic variety almost from the beginning of the illness *the right iliac fossa will appear empty on palpation,* owing to the taking up of the cæcum into the advancing invagination (Signe de Dance).

(8) *Constipation is by no means always absolute.* Exceptionally an intussusception may be present and yet the bowels may open fairly normally, and not uncommonly fæcal material may be mingled with the blood and mucus which come away. As the condition advances, however, the obstruction increases, and ultimately becomes absolute. One must therefore be prepared sometimes to diagnose intussusception in the absence of absolute constipation.

(9) As the intussusception approaches the rectum *tenesmus* may be indicated by the constant straining efforts of the infant. At this stage the congested apex may sometimes be felt on rectal examination.

(10) In late or neglected cases the increasing obstruction of the lumen of the gut results in *abdominal distension* and increased frequency of vomiting.

(11) In some cases the *apex* of the intussusception *may protrude through the anus* as a red congested fleshy mass.

(12) The final stage is that of complete intestinal obstruction, and peritonitis due to gangrene of the devitalized gut and infection of the peritoneum. Repeated vomiting, signs of toxæmia, and exhaustion end the scene.

In addition to the above symptoms fever up to 100° F. or even higher may be present as early as within the first 24 hours (Morrison and Court).

Diagnosis.—It is not usually difficult to diagnose an intussusception. The age of the child, the previous good health and sudden onset of acute pain coming on in bouts, which cause severe temporary shock, the passage of blood and mucus per rectum, and the presence of a sausage-shaped swelling in the abdomen are sufficiently characteristic to admit of no doubt. The cases of real doubt are those in which when the doctor sees the patient the attacks of pain may be quiescent and no tumour can be felt. In such cases, if the history is at all suggestive or characteristic, and blood and mucus have been passed, an anæsthetic may be given in order to examine the abdomen carefully for a lump. If an X-ray apparatus is available it is better to give a barium enema and take photographs. By this means the diagnosis can be definitely made, and at the same time the enema will help to reduce any intussusception which may be present. (See Fig. 27.)

Differential diagnosis.—In the early stages the condition must be distinguished from :

Simple colic.
Colitis.
Rectal polypus.

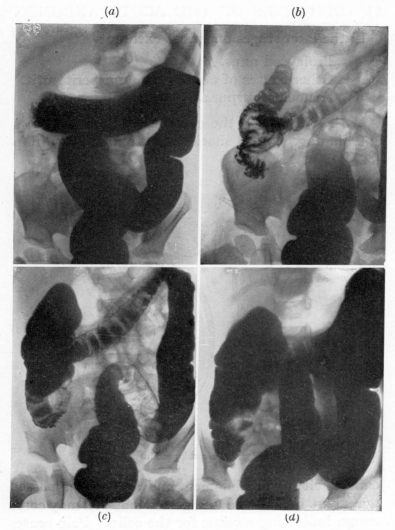

(a) $\qquad$ (b)

(c) $\qquad$ (d)

FIG. 27.—Series of radiograms taken during the administration of a barium enema in a case of intussusception.

(a) The opaque barium stopped its advance in the transverse colon at the site of the intussusception.

(b) The enema is reducing the intussusception and filling the ascending colon.

(c) The intussusception has been forced back to the cæcum which is filling with barium.

(d) There still remains a small part of the cæcum which does not fill with barium. Operation showed this was due to the last unreduced part of the intussusception.

In the later stages one must exclude :

Prolapsed anus.
Other causes of obstruction and peritonitis.
Henoch's purpura.

With *simple colic* the evidence of pain is not so outstanding, nor is shock so extreme. No lump

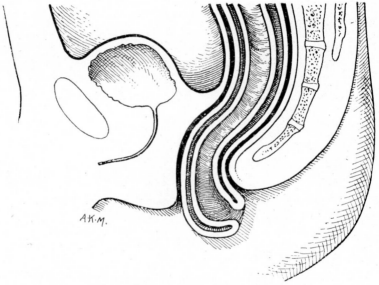

FIG. 28.—Diagram of prolapsed intussusception

can be felt in the abdomen, and no blood is passed per anum, but instead undigested material may come away, indicating a cause for the colic. Pain ceases when the bowels are emptied of the undigested or irritating contents.

Colitis and enterocolitis.—These furnish the main difficulty in diagnosis in young infants, amongst whom acute colitis is very common—especially in the autumn. Colitis is frequently accompanied by

the passage of blood and mucus per rectum.   The
chief distinguishing features are as follows :

(1) In colitis there is usually a stage of preliminary diarrhœa unaccompanied by blood.

(2) The infants who readily fall victims to
colitis are more frequently ill-nourished children.
Intussusception usually attacks well-nourished, fat
infants.

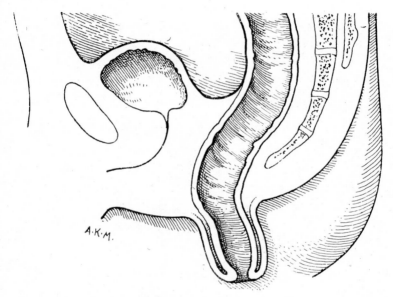

FIG. 29.—Diagram of rectal prolapse.

(3) In colitis there are more frequent stools, as a
rule containing more fæcal material than in cases
of intussusception.

(4) In colitis there is no abdominal tumour to be
felt, and

(5) The cæcum can be felt in the right iliac fossa,
and possibly gurgling may be elicited by pressing
on it.   There is not that emptiness which is so

noticeable on palpating the fossa in cases of intussusception.

(6) The crises of pain are not usually so severe in
colitis.

(7) In colitis there will sometimes be tenderness
along the whole course of the colon.

Obstructive symptoms and distension are not so
common in colitis. Tenesmus may be present in
both cases. There may be an epidemic of similar
cases which may help in the diagnosis of colitis. As
mentioned above, a radiograph after giving a barium
enema will always settle the diagnosis. Two or three
degrees of fever may be present in each condition
so this symptom cannot be used as a differentiating
help.

Cases in which the apex of the invagination
protrudes through the anus have to be distinguished from *prolapsus ani* (Figs. 28 and 29).
In the latter there is a ring of prolapsed mucous
membrane seen around a central opening, and the
finger or a probe cannot be inserted between the
mucosa and the external sphincter; in a prolapsed
intussusception the opening of the protruding
portion is towards the posterior aspect of the projection, and the finger can be inserted between the
anterior or lateral portions of the projection and
the anal sphincter. Any intussusception which has
advanced to the anus will be accompanied by considerable distension and symptoms of intestinal
obstruction.

The late stages of an intussusception of which
the apex has not advanced as far as the rectum,
and which is accompanied by advanced symptoms
of intestinal obstruction or peritonitis (i.e. disten-

sion, frequent vomiting, toxæmia, and collapse) can only be diagnosed from the other causes of those symptoms by the history of onset and previous course of the disease.

In children who have passed infancy, and occasionally in infants, intussusception has to be distinguished from *Henoch's purpura*, a disease characterized by abdominal pain, vomiting, the passage of blood per anum, and frequently accompanied by arthritis and an eruption of purpuric spots. The bleeding from the gut is due to an effusion of blood into the walls of the intestine. The youngest child in the series described by Henoch was four years old, so the age-incidence of the two diseases may be a help in diagnosis. In doubtful cases a very thorough search must be made for purpuric spots or for joint-affections. Very rarely the two conditions have been coexistent. Here again a barium enema may clinch the diagnosis.

In making a rectal examination of a child with an intussusception which has advanced to the descending or sigmoid colon, though it may be impossible to feel the swollen advancing apex, yet there may be characteristic œdema of the mucous membrane of the rectum in advance of the apex. There may be also a certain amount of ballooning of the rectum.

Subacute and chronic intussusception.—There are some cases of chronic intussusception which are accompanied by slight signs of intestinal obstruction, but progress steadily with repeated attacks of pain, sometimes at considerable intervals, until a final serious attack of obstruction occurs. Such cases are accompanied by but slight signs of intestinal obstruction, but progress steadily with repeated attacks of pain, sometimes at considerable intervals, until a final serious attack of obstruction occurs. In these cases there may be normal or almost normal fæcal motions until the final attack, and the observer is very likely to be misled by the chronicity or intermittence of the symptoms. I have known such a case taken for *tuberculous peritonitis and enteritis*. There were loose fæcal motions, and an epigastric swelling thought to be rolled-up omentum, but in reality an intussusception. In these subacute cases the help afforded by radiography after administration of a bismuth or barium meal is of the utmost value.

If after thorough examination there still remains doubt about the diagnosis of an intussusception, it should be regarded as less risky to advise exploration of the abdomen than to wait for serious acute obstructive symptoms.

Intussusception of pelvic colon in old people.— Intussusception is very rare in old people, but when it does occur generally affects the sigmoido-rectal region. This leads to frequent hypogastric pains and tenesmus, whilst mucus, and later blood, are passed through a rather patulous anus. Rectal examination easily demonstrates the œdematous apex of the intussusception, which is seldom more than a few inches long. A malignant growth may sometimes form the apex.

CHAPTER IX

CANCER OF THE LARGE BOWEL
VOLVULUS

IF strangulated hernia be excluded, cancer of the large bowel is the commonest cause of intestinal obstruction in persons over middle age. The symptoms are often insidious, and though in most cases an acute attack of obstruction may be the direct cause for the calling in of the surgeon, yet there are many earlier warning signs and symptoms which should put the observer on guard and cause a thorough examination to be made.

Early [1] diagnosis of cancer of the colon will lead to the prevention of obstruction by earlier treatment. For that purpose we consider it useful to include here a brief summary of the early symptoms.

The pathological character of the cancer may be either that of a rather quickly growing adeno-carcinoma or more commonly a scirrhus-type which contracts as it grows until a small tight stricture round the bowel is formed (Fig. 30). Glands are usually involved rather late, so that early diagnosis is desirable both to prevent obstruction and to permit a favourable attempt at cure.

The symptoms of cancer of the colon prior to an

[1] *Vide* Z. Cope, " Carcinoma of the Colon," *Brit. Med. Journ.*, 1912.

attack of acute obstruction may be considered under the following heads :

(1) *Symptoms due to bowel-ulceration.*

Diarrhœa and the passage of blood and mucus may result from ulceration of the bowel. The

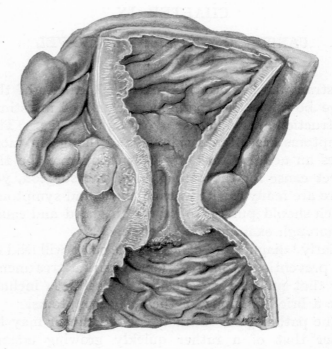

Fig. 30.—Drawing of the common ring-type of scirrhus-cancer of the colon which causes intestinal obstruction. (From a specimen in St. Mary's Hospital Museum.)

occurrence of diarrhœa may lead patients to assert that the bowels are regular, whereas the looseness is but secondary to the irritation caused by the constipated fæces. Owing to the presence of mucus the condition may wrongly be diagnosed mucous colitis.

(2) *The presence of a tumour*, which in the early stages may be freely mobile. This is uncommon, since the majority of the cases are of the contracting scirrhoid type with no palpable tumour.

(3) *Symptoms due to extension to other viscera.* The growth may adhere to the bladder, or pelvis of the kidney, and cause symptoms referable to the urinary organs, or may cause gastric symptoms owing to adhesion to the stomach.

(4) *Pericolitis*, or inflammation of the tissues round the colon, may be the first symptom of note. A local abscess may form and mask the primary condition. Sometimes perforation of the bowel suddenly takes place into the general peritoneal cavity, and diffuse and generally fatal peritonitis ensues.

(5) *Symptoms of subacute obstruction.*—These comprise the same symptoms as those caused by acute obstruction, but they are all of slighter degree. *Gradually increasing constipation* is often the first abnormality, and if this supervenes in a person over middle age who has previously been perfectly regular as to the bowels, suspicion should be aroused and thorough investigation carried out. Diarrhœa sometimes alternates with the constipation. Occasional attacks of distension and flatulence are common. Peristalsis may sometimes be seen through the abdominal wall, and local swelling may subside with a gurgling sound due to passage of flatus through the stricture. Pain is cramp-like and due to the peristalsis. Sometimes the patient will describe the pain as travelling across the abdomen and increasing in intensity up to the site where the gurgling occurs and where the obstruction is situated. The pain is often mistaken for indiges-

tion, and the accompanying nausea or sickness attributed to a bilious attack.

(6) *Acute obstruction* is sometimes the first signifi-cant symptom which compels attention. When acute symptoms supervene in a case of cancer of the colon it will sometimes be found that the ileo-cæcal valve has lost its efficiency so that the obstructive pressure is forced back into the small

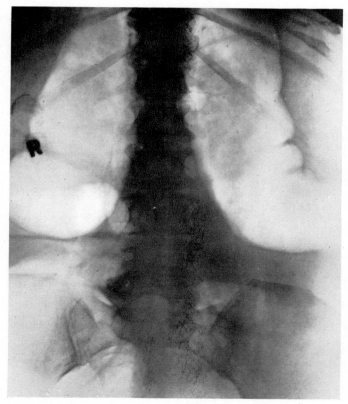

Fig. 31.—Plain X-ray of the abdomen of a patient suffering from obstruction of the colon. The cæcum, ascending colon, and descending colon are distended, but the distension stops abruptly in the region of the left iliac fossa, where the iliac colon was obstructed by a carcinoma.

gut. Very severe pain and frequent vomiting may then occur. When this happens it is frequently impossible to say what is the exact cause of the obstruction. In the case of both subacute and acute obstruction of the large bowel, either by carcinoma or by any other condition which narrows the lumen, great assistance in diagnosis can be gained by examination of a plain X-ray photograph. The distended part of the colon is as a rule clearly outlined, and frequently the position of the obstruction can be demonstrated at the site where the distended part of the bowel ceases. (Fig. 31.)

Distension, vomiting, pain, and constipation occurring in an elderly person, without any evidence of peritonitis, are generally due either to cancer of the large bowel, volvulus, diverticulitis, or very rarely to intussusception or uræmia. Rectal examination to detect a cancer of the rectum and lower sigmoid, and examination of the urine to exclude chronic renal disease, are both necessary procedures. The symptoms of subacute volvulus are not always distinguishable from those of chronic stricture of the bowel.

Diverticulitis, when it causes a stricture, produces symptoms undistinguishable from those of carcinoma of the bowel.

Volvulus of the large intestine occurs in two places —the sigmoid and the cæcal regions. The sigmoid is by far the most common situation, owing to the fact that the sigmoid meso-colon is long and the base of attachment narrow, so that twisting of the loop more readily occurs. Ileo-cæcal volvulus is more rare.

Sigmoid volvulus causes symptoms of acute or

subacute intestinal obstruction of large bowel type. There is usually a preliminary period during which attacks of abdominal pain and constipation may occur.

The *acute attack* is signalized by absolute constipation (very quickly demonstrated by administering a turpentine enema), acute abdominal pain, and

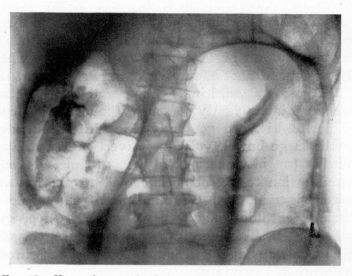

Fig. 32.—X-ray photograph of sigmoid volvulus showing enormous distension of the coil which extends up to the left hypochondrium.

rapid distension of the abdomen. (According to Barnard the early appearance of tenderness due to onset of peritonitis is a distinguishing feature, but this would only follow quickly where there was an absolute strangulation of the coil, which is by no means constant.) If the vessels of the loop are completely occluded gangrene of the loop quickly occurs, and peritonitis ensues rapidly. The great abdominal distension may seriously impede respiration.

Subacute sigmoid volvulus is distinguished by abdominal pain (chiefly referred to the umbilical and hypogastric zones), constipation, and gradually increasing distension. The distended sigmoid coil may stand out sometimes in the lower abdomen like the segment of a large pneumatic tyre, but later the whole abdomen will become generally distended.

Though the diagnosis of volvulus is not always made before operation the condition should be suspected when early and great distension supervenes in a case of acute obstruction. Localization of the distension to the hypogastrium at the outset, or the standing out of one large coil, may point clearly to a sigmoid volvulus. Though the pain of sigmoid volvulus is usually hypogastric and not severe, I have known a twisted sigmoid in a young woman cause such severe pain in the lower lumbar region posteriorly that it was thought the pain might be due to acute dysmenorrhœa.

Considerable help can be gained from examination of a plain X-ray of the abdomen when the one distended coil may be plainly visible. (See X-ray, p. 158.) Volvulus of the transverse colon is seldom seen except after major abdominal operations in which the intestines have had to be displaced and the colon may have been twisted in replacement.

Ileo-cœcal volvulus gives rise to symptoms similar to, but more acute than, those described under obstruction of the lower end of the small gut, but in addition there will be a localized distension due to the dilated cæcum, observable either in the epigastrium or the right side of the abdomen. Pain is very severe and vomiting is a prominent symptom.

Later, the general distension would mask the local cæcal dilatation.

Differential diagnosis of obstruction of the large gut. —In every case it is necessary first to examine all the hernial apertures.

There are four conditions which may deceive the observer and cause him erroneously to believe that he is dealing with a case of primary obstruction of the large bowel.   They are :

(1) **Colitis with distension.**
(2) **Uræmia.**
(3) **Peritonitis.**
(4) **Reflex paralysis of colon.**

Colitis with atonic distension of the inflamed bowel. —There are cases of severe ulcerative colitis in which either as a direct result of the ulceration or as a consequence of the toxæmia the large bowel becomes enormously distended and atonic, so that organic obstruction is diagnosed.   If seen at a late stage for the first time it may be impossible to distinguish between the two conditions, but the long history of symptoms pointing to ulceration of the colon (diarrhœa, with passage of blood and mucus) in the one case, and the usual history of subacute obstruction in the other, may help in determining.   In ulcerative colitis the obstruction is never complete and an enema will bring away flatus, whilst the toxic symptoms will be greater. If seen at an earlier stage a radiograph taken after a bismuth or barium meal might demonstrate any obstruction in the colon, but the patients are often too ill to have this done.

Uræmia.—Abdominal distension and vomiting are sometimes seen in uræmia, and unless a practice is made of examining the urine for albumin in every case of supposed intestinal obstruction in middle-aged or older persons, serious mistakes will be made. The estimation of the blood-pressure and the percussion of the cardiac dullness may throw light on doubtful cases. Symptoms indistinguishable from those of intestinal obstruction may occur in acute nephritis, chronic nephritis, and fibro-cystic disease of the kidneys.

Peritonitis.—There are some forms of peritonitis which are accompanied by very slight rigidity of the abdominal wall, and there are some abdominal walls in fat, flabby subjects which are almost incapable of becoming rigid on account of the weak and fat-infiltrated muscles. In such patients the distension and vomiting of peritonitis may be mistaken for mechanical obstruction. The late stages of peritonitis are accompanied by a paralytic obstruction of the bowels, and the later stages of intestinal obstruction are frequently accompanied by peritonitis, due to organisms escaping through patches of local gangrene or malnutrition of the gut.

In the early stage of both conditions diagnosis is usually clear on considering the history and symptoms, but in the later stages it may be impossible to differentiate.

Reflex paralysis of the colon.—There is a deceptive form of paralytic distension of the colon which on several occasions I have known to simulate obstruction of the large bowel. It appears to be a reflex result of an acute inflammation somewhere in the abdomen, and in three cases which I can recall was a secondary effect of acute cholecystitis, and masked the primary condition. The ascending, transverse, and descending colon may be distended, and it may be difficult to get the bowels to act These symptoms, with the pain and vomiting, are sufficient to divert from the true cause unless special care be taken.

CHAPTER X

THE EARLY DIAGNOSIS OF STRANGULATED AND OBSTRUCTED HERNIÆ

A STRANGULATED hernia is one of the most dangerous forms of intestinal obstruction. The hernial orifices through which the abdominal contents protrude have for the most part hard fibrous edges which quickly either cause local necrosis of the gut at the site of pressure, or cause interference with the blood-supply in the accompanying mesentery with consequent gangrene of the gut. It is often very difficult to make certain whether a hernia is merely obstructed or whether it is strangulated, for pain and constipation are usually present in both cases.

The symptoms of a strangulated hernia are those of intestinal obstruction with the addition of a painful, tender, and often tense swelling in one of the hernial regions The type of obstructive symptoms will naturally vary according to the part of the gut obstructed in the sac. If jejunum be caught in the hernia very acute symptoms ensue, if ileum be obstructed less acute manifestations result, whilst with large bowel alone in the sac the symptoms are usually subacute but none the less serious. When omentum alone is strangulated there will be pain, constipation, nausea, and sometimes vomiting, but the obstruction is never complete and the bowels may be emptied by enemata.

Shock is a variable factor, but may be very acute in some strangulations. The vomiting gradually becomes fæculent when gut is strangled.

Since, apart from operation, it is next to impossible to make certain that there is no gut in the sac, and inasmuch as mechanical obstruction to the bowel is ultimately as dangerous as strangulation, it is well to treat all painful tense herniæ as if they were strangulated. We consider that, save in the case of very easily reducible swellings, all painful herniæ, accompanied by abdominal pain and other symptoms of obstruction, should be treated as strangulated herniæ by operation without attempting taxis. If an anæsthetic has to be given for reduction it is much better to reduce by open operation. Fomentations and icebags should be regarded as causing unwise and dangerous delay, and taxis should only be adopted when surgical operative procedures are for good reasons impossible.

There are a few practical diagnostic points which may be considered with each of the several varieties of hernia.

STRANGULATED INGUINAL HERNIA

It is usually a very easy matter to diagnose a strangulated inguinal hernia. The patient has usually been aware of the existence of the hernia for some time, and may have been wearing a truss. The sudden coming down of the rupture, accompanied by abdominal pain, vomiting, and tenseness and tenderness in the local swelling, make a clear picture. But mistakes are possible in the following conditions :

An inflamed hernia may cause local symptoms

similar to those present in one that is strangulated, but shock is absent, intra-abdominal pain is absent or slight, and vomiting is quite a minor feature and never becomes fæculent.

Acute hydrocele of the cord, though rare, has been known to simulate a strangulated hernia, but the painful tense inguinal swelling of an acute hydrocele would not cause so severe vomiting and never fæculent vomiting, nor would there be any evidence of intestinal obstruction. Turpentine enemata would always produce a satisfactory result.

Vomiting due to some other condition may in the presence of an unreduced inguinal hernia give rise to a suspicion of strangulation. The vomiting of pregnancy or that at the onset of appendicitis may lead to this mistake. But in such cases the sac is usually neither tender nor tense, and the contents may be easily reducible. When a catastrophe, such as the perforation of an ulcer or rupture of the gall bladder, happens to occur in a patient who has an unreduced hernia, there will be tenderness over the hernial site, and diagnosis has to be made by considering the history and other abdominal signs and symptoms.

Inflamed inguinal or iliac glands.—With these the swelling is usually more diffuse and fixed, and there are redness and œdema of the skin and subcutaneous tissues. Vomiting and intra-abdominal pain will be absent or slight, and fever is sure to be present.

Torsion or inflammation of an inguinal testis may occasionally closely simulate a strangulated hernia. The absence of the testicle from the scrotum on the affected side should make one consider the possibility of the condition. In torsion of the testicle the local pain is very severe, and vomiting will begin early in the case but never become fæculent. Though constipation may be a symptom, enemata will produce satisfactory results.

When a metastasis of mumps occurs in an inguinal testis—a very rare occurrence—it might lead to a diagnosis of strangulated hernia, but there would be no intestinal obstruction.

It is to be remembered that a retained testis is often associated with a hernia of the interstitial variety.

Thrombosis or suppurative phlebitis of the veins of the spermatic cord causes a painful swelling of the cord and its surroundings, but with these conditions the testicle is swollen and tender and will give the clue to the condition.

On several occasions I have known a subperitoneal fibroid in pregnant women to cause a swelling in the inguinal region, and lead to suspicion of strangulated hernia on account of the coincident vomiting of pregnancy. Careful examination enables one to feel the tumour move separately from the abdominal wall, and, of course, the vomiting never becomes fæculent and the tumour is not usually tender.

STRANGULATED FEMORAL HERNIA

A strangulated femoral hernia gives rise to more mistakes in diagnosis than a strangulated inguinal hernia. The hernia is often very small and may easily escape notice in the thick fat often present in the saphenous region. Sometimes only a small knuckle of gut comprising but a small portion of the circumference of the bowel may be caught in the crural canal, and scarcely any projection may be felt in the thigh. When the hernia is of a large size it consists of a rounded fundus and a narrow neck or stalk which permits free and often *painless* side-to-side movement of the fundal part. This absence of fixity of the sac may lead the observer to think that there is no strangulation.

A strangulated femoral hernia might be simulated by (1) an inflamed inguinal gland, (2) thrombosis of a saphenous varix, (3) an inflamed appendix in a femoral hernial sac, (4) a tense and painful hydrocele of a femoral hernial sac, whilst (5) a strangulated inguinal hernia has often been wrongly diagnosed when a femoral sac was causing the trouble.

An **inflamed gland** is usually more fixed, gives rise to more œdema and possibly redness of the parts overlying, and usually results from a primary cause which may be detected on the corresponding thigh or ano-perineal region. Vomiting and intestinal obstruction are, of course, absent.

A **thrombosed saphenous varix** would not ordinarily give rise to vomiting or abdominal pain. If the thrombosis extends up to the iliac vein there will be pain and tenderness in the iliac region.

An **inflamed appendix in a femoral hernial sac** cannot be distinguished definitely from a strangulated omental femoral hernia before operation, though by the history of previous attacks of appendicitis it might be suspected. If fæculent vomiting occur it would, of course, be clear that bowel was strangled in the sac. The presence of an inflamed appendix would be suspected if hyperæsthesia were elicited within the iliac triangular area.

A **strangulated inguinal hernia** must be distinguished by noting that the swelling comes out of the abdomen medially to the pubic spine and above Poupart's ligament.

In general, any swelling in the region of the femoral canal which suddenly appears or becomes larger and more painful, and is accompanied by vomiting *or nausea*, should be considered as a case of femoral hernia in need of immediate operation.

In those rare cases in which a pouch of the cæcum becomes tightly gripped in a femoral hernia, there may be no abdominal pain, no vomiting and no intestinal obstruction, even though the herniated portion become gangrenous. This fact makes it all the more necessary to explore any doubtful tender lump in the femoral region.

OBSTRUCTED AND STRANGULATED UMBILICAL AND VENTRAL HERNIÆ

Umbilical or para-umbilical hernia is most common in women, and chiefly seen in fat persons. A very fat woman in a surgical ward is nearly always there on account of gall-stones or an umbilical hernia.

An umbilical hernia usually contains omentum and frequently large bowel. Small intestine is not quite so commonly found in the sac. When obstruction or strangulation occurs the symptoms are therefore much more likely to be subacute, and partake more of the character of large-bowel obstruction. The two common mistakes made in regard to umbilical hernia are (1) to overlook a small hernia lying deeply embedded in fat, and (2) to think that the hernia is not strangulated because the symptoms are not very acute. The fact that the mortality for operations on strangulated umbilical hernia is three times that for strangulated inguinal and femoral shows the serious need for more early diagnosis and interference.

It is quite common for a patient to have several attacks of obstruction before the more serious strangulation-attack occurs. The fact that on previous occasions the obstruction has been overcome by aperients may lead to an erroneous opinion that the same will occur again. The symptoms of the two conditions are at first similar. It is sometimes only by the most serious symptoms of strangulation (gangrene of gut or omentum, fæcal abscess, even gangrene of the skin overlying the hernia) that the patient and medical attendant

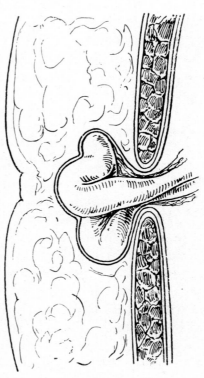

FIG. 33.—Drawing to show how an umbilical hernia may be embedded in and hidden by a fat abdominal wall.

realize the extremely serious nature of the case.

The diagnosis of an obstructed umbilical hernia is made on the occurrence of abdominal pain, vomiting, constipation, and local tenderness on pressure over the swelling, which can always be felt deep in

the fat, even if it does not bulge obviously on the
surface in the region of the umbilicus. The administration of two turpentine enemata, with an interval
of a few hours, will determine whether real obstruction of the large bowel exists, and if that is demonstrated it is unwise to wait for the more serious
symptoms of strangulation before advising operation.
If small gut be obstructed in the sac symptoms will
be correspondingly more acute and vomiting will
soon become fæculent.

It is often difficult to say before opening the sac
whether one is dealing with simple obstruction or
with strangulation.

Ventral hernia.—The same general remarks apply
here as in the case of umbilical hernia, with the
exception that small bowel is more commonly
found in the sac, and consequently acute symptoms
are more frequently observed. Abdominal pain,
vomiting, constipation, and local tenderness over
the site of a ventral hernia are sufficient to indicate
the need for operation.

Obturator hernia is very rare and should be
classed among the internal herniæ, since there is
usually no external swelling, though there may be
tenderness and a little fullness in the upper adductor
region of the corresponding thigh. The condition
is rarely diagnosed before opening the abdomen, but
it is possible that the thigh-rotation test might give
assistance in diagnosis.

CHAPTER XI

ACUTE ABDOMINAL SYMPTOMS IN PREGNANCY AND THE PUERPERIUM

ACUTE abdominal pain in a pregnant woman is always a source of special anxiety, both from the maternal and the fœtal point of view. Exploratory operations are not lightly to be advised on account of the risk of abortion, and one therefore needs to be very sure of the indications of the various acute diseases needing intervention before advising the abdomen to be opened.

The following conditions giving rise to acute abdominal symptoms may be met with during pregnancy or the puerperium:

   (1) Persistent vomiting.
   (2) Ectopic pregnancy.
   (3) Retroverted gravid uterus.
   (4) Threatened abortion.
   (5) Sepsis following attempts at abortion.
   (6) Pyelitis.
   (7) Degeneration in a fibroid.
   (8) Spontaneous rupture of the uterus.
   (9) Appendicitis.
  (10) Perforated gastric ulcer.
  (11) Torsion of the pedicle of an ovarian cyst or pedunculated fibroid, or torsion of a normal ovary.
  (12) Pelvic peritonitis or cellulitis.

171

Persistent vomiting.—The morning vomiting of pregnancy usually begins in the second and continues through the third month. As a rule it does not cause any anxiety, but when accompanied by any abnormality in the abdomen it may give rise to doubt. On several occasions I have known serious doubt occur in pregnant women who were vomiting and also had a slightly painful swelling in the right inguinal region. It was thought that a strangulated inguinal hernia might be causing the symptoms, but examination showed in each case a uterine fibroid which had risen out of the pelvis with the enlarging uterus and had simulated a hernia by bulging out the inguinal canal. The vomiting in such cases takes place without reference to any pain in the swelling, and it is possible to feel any intra-abdominal swelling move independently of the abdominal wall on deep respiration.

I have also known the vomiting of early pregnancy, when accompanied by slight pelvic pain due to congestion or constipation, to be mistaken for appendicitis, but careful pelvic and abdominal examination, and a close attention to the symptom-sequence, should exclude this condition.

The excessive vomiting due to the toxæmia of pregnancy does not concern us here, but it is necessary to make sure that there is not any serious intra-abdominal lesion before diagnosing hyperemesis gravidarum.

Ectopic pregnancy is so important and common that the next chapter is devoted to that subject alone.

A retroverted gravid uterus, or, as it was well termed by Matthews Duncan, " the disease of the third and fourth months of pregnancy," may give rise to acute abdominal pain felt chiefly in the hypogastrium, where the distended bladder is situated. The fact of pregnancy considered along with the presence of a hypogastric swelling (larger than the uterus should be for that time of gestation), the occurrence of pain, nausea, and retention of urine (or maybe dribbling incontinence), would cause one to suspect the condition, which would be easily diagnosed after the urine had been drawn off.

Threatened abortion should cause no difficulty in diagnosis when pregnancy is known to exist, since the uterine bleeding with the lumbar backache and hypogastric pain, and the absence of evidence of any other local abnormality, should sufficiently determine the condition.

Sepsis following attempt to produce abortion.—It is unfortunately not unknown for women to try either to produce abortion on themselves or to persuade some lay person to attempt a similar disservice for them. Sepsis may follow these attempts, and when the doctor is called in it may be difficult to obtain any history of interference. The sepsis may take the form of a peritonitis, a septicæmia, or both. There is generally bleeding from the uterus. In any case, therefore, of bleeding from the uterus in a woman who has had a period of amenorrhœa and in whom abdominal pain, vomiting, and fever suddenly present themselves, one must bear in mind the possibility of uterine sepsis. Septicæmia and peritonitis in such cases are usually rapid and virulent. The onset is unlike that of any other abdominal condition, and the pain may not only be felt in the hypogastrium but may be referred to the back or down the legs.   Careful bimanual examination will determine an enlarged softened uterus and may exclude any other pelvic condition.   In any such case it is wise to have a consultation with a fellow-practitioner before deciding on any course of action.

Pyelitis is not an uncommon complication of pregnancy.   It occurs usually about the fourth month of gestation, and its onset may have some relationship to the pressure of the growing uterus upon the ureters, especially the right ureter, for the condition is more common on the right side.

The symptoms commonly start with a rigor or feeling of chilliness, and the temperature quickly rises to 103° F. or thereabouts.   At the same time pain is felt in one or other loin (generally the right) under the costal margin.   Pressure at the erector-costal angle produces pain.   There may be some frequency of and pain on micturition, but this is not constant.   There is as a rule no rigidity of abdominal muscles.   In some cases the patient does not feel ill, whilst at other times there may be severe malaise.   Examination of the urine shows turbidity, albuminuria, and the presence of pus in small quantity.   Bacteria (usually *bacillus coli communis*) will be detected on microscopical examination.   The albumin may not be more than is to be expected to correspond with the pus.

When on the right side differential diagnosis must be made from appendicitis.   This is usually easy, for appendicitis seldom starts with a rigor, infrequently causes such high fever as 103° or 104° F., and is often accompanied by local rigidity, and not so frequently by any urinary trouble.   Examination of the urine should settle the diagnosis.

Appendicitis and *perforated gastric ulcer* are misfortunes that may overtake the pregnant as any other woman, and they should be diagnosable readily by considering the symptoms carefully. Sometimes when they occur in the puerperium they may be mistaken for the results of puerperal sepsis. The symptoms, however, should be readily interpreted if the possibility of their occurrence be borne in mind.

In the puerperium also it is not uncommon for a dermoid or other *ovarian cyst* to become *inflamed* or undergo *torsion*, owing to the contusion and displacement consequent on the labour. There will be acute abdominal pain, fever, vomiting, and a tender hypogastrium, whilst a rounded swelling will be felt near the uterus but separate from it. A distended bladder should be excluded by catheterization, and a twisted fibroid by noting the relation to the uterus.

A slightly enlarged but otherwise normal ovary has been known to undergo torsion in early pregnancy and cause pain and vomiting so that an ectopic gestation was thought a likely diagnosis until the abdomen had been opened (Searle).

Red degeneration or necrobiosis of a uterine fibroid is particularly prone to occur during pregnancy. The symptoms are pain felt locally in the fibroid, which can be palpated through the abdominal wall, slight fever, and nausea or vomiting. In any patient who is known to have a fibroid and to be pregnant such symptoms would point to red degeneration, and in such cases it is sometimes possible for the fibroid to be enucleated without disturbing the pregnancy.

Spontaneous rupture of the pregnant uterus is a very rare condition leading to severe shock and signs of internal hæmorrhage. For details one must consult an obstetrical textbook.

Pelvic peritonitis may ensue after childbirth. Sometimes this may be septic in nature, but quite commonly it may be of gonorrhœal origin. Any vaginal discharge in the patient or the presence of infection of the baby's conjunctival sacs might give the clue. Hypogastric pain and tenderness, vomiting or nausea, and bilateral tenderness in the uterine fornices will be demonstrable.

ACUTE ABDOMINAL DISEASE PECULIAR TO WOMEN APART FROM PREGNANCY

Acute salpingitis.—Acute salpingitis is most commonly due to infection with the gonococcus. Another frequent cause is infection with the staphylococcus or streptococcus. It can also be caused by the *bacillus coli communis* (*Escherichia coli*) or the pneumococcus.

Symptoms and signs.—The picture is that of an attack of pelvic peritonitis—hypogastric pain, nausea or vomiting, and fever which may reach as high as 103°. Examination shows tenderness on pressure in both iliac fossæ and in the suprapubic region. In some cases the lower abdomen is rigid and moves badly on respiration, and there may be considerable distension. Vulval examination may show traces of a gonococcal infection, or a purulent vaginal discharge may be present. Palpation in the lateral fornices may cause pain.

Diagnosis.—The common and chief difficulty is to distinguish appendicitis from salpingitis (see Chapter V).

The symptom-sequence is usually more charac-

teristic in appendicitis, and the pain often more
strictly limited to the right side. In salpingitis
it is common for the pain to be worse on the left
side than on the right—an occurrence but rarely
seen in the *early* stages of appendicitis.

A vaginal discharge in which gonococci are
detected would be significant.

It is frequently very difficult and almost impossible to make quite certain whether the appendix
or salpinx is primarily at fault.

When pelvic peritonitis follows childbirth it may
not show itself for a week or more after the birth.

Pyosalpinx.—Many cases of salpingitis quieten
down and form a local collection of pus within
the Fallopian tube—pyosalpinx. The condition
is usually bilateral. For a time symptoms may
abate and be almost negligible, but sooner or
later the infection spreads and an extension of
inflammation occurs. There will be the symptoms
of pelvic peritonitis as in the case of salpingitis,
but in addition there will be felt a bilateral tender
swelling in the pouch of Douglas. The symptoms
in a ruptured pyosalpinx are often the more serious
since there is frequently secondary infection of the
pus-sac by organisms other than the gonococcus.

An ovarian cyst with twisted pedicle gives rise to
acute symptoms. Hypogastric pain, vomiting, and
the presence of a tender swelling in the lower
abdomen are the principal features.

The vomiting comes on almost as soon as the pain,
so that there is less likely to be an interval between
the initial pain and the vomiting as is usual in
appendicitis. With an ovarian cyst there will be a
definite, rounded, tender swelling to be felt either by

palpating the hypogastrium or by pelvic examination. If the case be not seen early, peritonitis with accompanying rigidity may prevent the full outline of the tumour being felt, and it may be difficult to distinguish from other causes of pelvic peritonitis, e.g. acute salpingitis with serous effusion, but the symptoms of a twisted ovarian cyst are usually the more acute.

Torsion of pedicle of hydrosalpinx.—With this the symptoms are similar to those of an ovarian cyst with twisted pedicle, though usually slighter in degree: pain, nausea or vomiting, and a tender, movable swelling in one or other vaginal fornix. In the presence of even the slightest menstrual irregularity it would be impossible certainly to exclude an unruptured ectopic gestation.

Rupture of an ovarian endometrioma may cause hypogastric pain, vomiting, and fever ; bimanual examination will reveal a swelling on one or both sides of the pouch of Douglas. This clinical picture might easily be mistaken for tubo-ovarian inflammation or even for pelvic appendicitis, and it would as a rule be difficult to make certain before exploration.

In every doubtful case of acute abdominal disease in women it is necessary to pass a catheter to make sure that the bladder is empty before making a final decision.

CHAPTER XII

ECTOPIC GESTATION

By ectopic gestation is meant the development of a fertilized ovum in any place other than the uterine cavity. The rupture of such a gestation sac is a comparatively common occurrence with fairly characteristic symptoms, yet it is often misdiagnosed.

Fertilization of the ovum probably normally takes place in the Fallopian tube, and any slight cause may detain the developing ovum, prevent its further progress and lead to an ectopic gestation. A fertilized ovum has been known very rarely to develop in the substance of the ovary, but this condition is of little practical importance, since one cannot clinically distinguish it. The commonest place for ectopic development of the ovum is in the ampullary part of the Fallopian tube. More rarely it is found in the isthmial part of the tube, and more rarely still it may develop in the tubo-uterine section of the tube, or in a rudimentary cornu, which for clinical purposes must be included in the same group (Fig. 34).

In a tubal gestation growth of the ovum leads to distension of the tube, whilst the eroding action of the villi leads to a thinning of the wall. Gradual oozing of blood may take place into the peritoneal cavity from the eroded area, or any sudden strain may lead to rupture of the tube.   Sometimes the

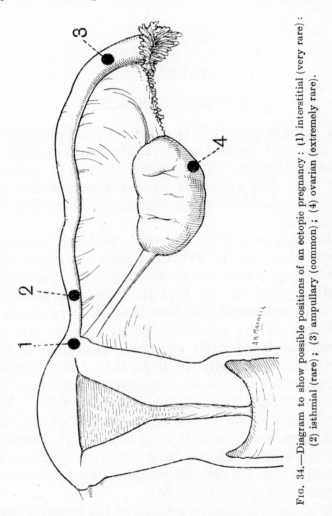

FIG. 34.—Diagram to show possible positions of an ectopic pregnancy : (1) interstitial (very rare) : (2) isthmial (rare) ; (3) ampullary (common) ; (4) ovarian (extremely rare).

ovum is extruded through the end of the tube into the peritoneal cavity by a process well termed " tubal abortion," or the embryo may die in consequence of hæmorrhage into the sac, or rupture of the sac into the lumen of the tube, and thus may be formed a tubal mole.

If the embryo lives, primary rupture of the sac occurs usually within the first eight weeks of pregnancy, though in the case of a tubo-uterine or interstitial gestation-sac rupture need not occur till pregnancy has advanced to the third or fourth month.

Rupture of the sac causes acute abdominal symptoms which usually subside with the formation of a collection of blood-clot in the pouch of Douglas (pelvic hæmatocele), but in some cases death may rapidly occur from the great internal hæmorrhage. It is exceptional for the sac to rupture into the broad ligament.

If the fœtus continues to develop after primary rupture of the tube severe symptoms may be caused at a later date by secondary rupture into the general peritoneal cavity.

Ectopic gestation often results from the first conception of a woman who has been married some years, or in a parous woman who has not been pregnant for several years.

Symptoms and diagnosis.—A patient with an ectopic gestation may seek advice for abdominal pain :

    (1) Before the sac has ruptured.
    (2) At the time of primary rupture of the sac.
    (3) Some days or even weeks after the rupture.

(1) Symptoms and diagnosis before the sac has ruptured.

If the serious complications ensuing on the rupture of a gestation-sac are to be avoided it is essential that the condition should, if possible, be diagnosed before the tube has given way. Sometimes there are few if any symptoms premonitory of rupture, but frequently there are indications of value which enable one to make a diagnosis with sufficient probability. There was a time when it was a rarity to diagnose and remove an inflamed appendix before it ruptured, now it is considered something of a reproach to allow an appendix to perforate before surgical advice is obtained. In like manner though not to the same degree it is likely that in the future greater attention will be paid to the correct diagnosis and operative treatment of a tubal pregnancy before primary rupture has occurred.

In a typical case (such as is seldom seen) the symptoms and signs would be :

> Amenorrhœa (for one or two months).
> Hypogastric pain.
> Uterine bleeding.
> Local hypogastric tenderness on pressing into pelvis toward one side.
> Small tender swelling in the lateral fornix.
> The passage of a membrane per vaginam.

Amenorrhœa.—Though in type-cases one or two periods may have been missed, the breasts may be slightly enlarged and full, and even sickness in the morning noted, yet such definite symptoms are rather exceptional.

There is, however, nearly always some slight

irregularity of menstruation, and care must be taken to ascertain exact particulars as to that event. The patient must be asked (1) when was the last period ; (2) if that period was before or after the normal time, noting a delay or advancement of as short a period as a day in women who are usually regular to the day ; (3) whether the loss at the last period was less or more than usual ; (4) whether any slight loss has occurred since the last regular period.

Since the gestation-sac of an embryo under a month old may rupture, or abort through the end of the tube, it is not absolutely necessary for there to be any irregularity of menstruation. Not uncommonly the bleeding from the vagina which accompanies tubal abortion is mistaken by the patient for the normal menstrual period, for it may coincide exactly with the expected menstruation. Usually the loss is less or greater than normal, and is antedated or postdated to the regular period by a day or several days. Sometimes what was apparently a normal period ceases for a few days, and then bleeding recommences. All these slight irregularities need to be noted.

Abdominal pain felt chiefly in the hypogastric or iliac regions may be the chief complaint. Taken in conjunction with the vaginal bleeding these pains may suggest both to patient and doctor a threatening abortion. The pains are probably due to repeated slight intra-peritoneal hæmorrhage, or to the contractions of the Fallopian tube.

Uterine bleeding has been referred to above. It is not constant. The blood as it comes away from the vagina is stated to be darker than the normal menstrual loss, but this is not of much value in diagnosis. What is of greater importance, if it occurs, is the passage of a decidual cast of the interior of the uterus. This seldom occurs till the embryo is dead, or aborted into the abdominal cavity, and often occurs after the operation for removal of a ruptured sac has been performed. If it occurs at the time of the early griping pains it is of the greatest importance in diagnosis. The shreds of membrane do not show any chorionic villi, and can thus be distinguished from an embryonal uterine sac. They should be floated out in water, so that the full size and shape may be ascertained.

Hypogastric tenderness may be detected on the side of the lesion if the fingers are gently pressed well down behind the pubis. The abdominal wall is not rigid.

Bimanual examination reveals a small rounded tender movable swelling to one side of the uterus in one or other lateral fornix corresponding to the side where the pain and tenderness are elicited. The uterus will also be felt slightly enlarged.

To sum up : if the patient and the doctor think that pregnancy has begun, if there be irregular hypogastric pain more on one side than the other, and if with slight uterine bleeding a tender rounded movable lump be felt to one side of a slightly enlarged uterus, ectopic pregnancy should be diagnosed and operation strongly advised. On one occasion when on such grounds I had diagnosed extra-uterine pregnancy and advised operation, the patient went for confirmation of the diagnosis to a hospital. Whilst waiting in the out-patient department of the hospital she collapsed from internal bleeding and had to be operated on promptly. It is

possible and should be a more frequent occurrence
to diagnose the condition before great internal
hæmorrhage occurs.

Differential diagnosis.—Grandin, in reference to
tubal gestation, observes : " The man who suspects
every woman of having the condition is the man
who is least liable to err in diagnosis." It is frequently misdiagnosed because infrequently considered. An early unruptured tubal pregnancy
needs to be distinguished from :

> **Gastritis.**
> **Appendicitis.**
> **Threatened uterine abortion.**
> **Pyo- or hydrosalpinx.**
> **Small ovarian or broad ligament cysts.**

It is only by the casual observer who has not
examined the patient that the colicky pain of an
ectopic pregnancy threatening to rupture can be
mistaken for gastritis. The position and nature
of the pain should direct attention to the pelvis,
where examination will soon provide facts for
correct diagnosis.

If the gestation be in the right tube it is easily
mistaken for *appendicitis*. Some of the main
points in diagnosis may be tabulated :

	Symptoms of an unruptured inflamed pelvic appendix.	Symptoms due to an unruptured (but possibly leaking) tubal gestation.
Menstruation.	Usually regular.	Usually some irregularity.
Uterine bleeding.	Usually none.	Usually present.
Initial pain.	Epigastric.	Hypogastric.
Fever.	Slight fever.	Usually no fever.
Vomiting or nausea.	Present.	Unusual.
Bimanual examination.	Tenderness but no movable lump.	A tender rounded movable swelling to one side of the uterus.

If the appendix is not situated in the pelvis there can be little likelihood of mistake. Neither with a pelvic appendicitis nor with a tubal gestation is there, as a rule, any rigidity of the abdominal wall.

A threatened uterine abortion is often difficult to distinguish, and on several occasions I have known uterine curettage performed for what was thought to be an incomplete abortion, but was in reality a tubal gestation. Bimanual examination ought to distinguish, for if it be definitely decided that pregnancy has begun, and there be uterine bleeding, pelvic examination will show in the one case a slightly enlarged uterus with a small swelling to one side, and in the other case a larger uterus with no swelling in the lateral fornix.

The greatest difficulty in diagnosis would be in the case of an intra-uterine pregnancy complicated by a pyosalpinx, hydrosalpinx, or small ovarian cyst. If severe abdominal pain occurred with any of these it might be impossible to diagnose with certainty, but abdominal section would probably be indicated in any case.

(2) Symptoms and diagnosis at the time of rupture or tubal abortion with profuse intra-peritoneal bleeding.

Rupture of a tubal gestation is probably the commonest cause of sudden death in young women who have previously been in perfect health. It brings many more to the gates of death.

The symptoms are usually clear :

> Sudden abdominal pain.
> Vomiting.
> Faintness or actual fainting.

Sudden anæmia and collapse with small
rapid pulse and subnormal temperature.
A tender tumid abdomen.
Free fluid in abdominal cavity.
Tenderness on pressing finger against Doug-
las' pouch.

The pain is sometimes hypogastric, sometimes
more general or even epigastric ; occasionally pain
is felt over the clavicles or even in the supra-spinous
fossa. The anæmia should be looked for especially
in the lips, tongue, and under the finger-nails. The
sclerotics also have a particularly white appearance,
and there is sometimes a dark ring round the eyes.
Restlessness and occasional deep sighing respirations
may indicate the severe internal hæmorrhage.

The pulse-rate is by no means always a good guide
as to the bleeding, for in some people it takes a
very large hæmorrhage to cause much increase in
rapidity, and in others rapid compensation and
restoration of the circulation occur. Nevertheless
the pulse is usually rapid and very feeble, and the
blood-pressure is often considerably lowered.

Examination of the abdomen will show a flaccid
but tender abdomen, with some fullness and (exceptionally) slight resistance to palpation in the
hypogastrium. Free fluid may be demonstrated,
but it is unnecessary and unwise to do so. The
pelvic peritoneum will be tender and a swelling may
possibly be detectable in one lateral fornix. The
important points to pay attention to are the sudden
onset, the fainting attack, the grave anæmia, feeble
pulse, and subnormal temperature.

Differential diagnosis must be made from several
of the very acute abdominal catastrophes, such as

perforation of the stomach, duodenum, or gall-
bladder, acute intestinal obstruction, acute pancreatitis, acute perforative appendicitis, or torsion
of the pedicle of an ovarian cyst. The history of
the case, the sudden onset and the persistence of
the extreme pallor and subnormal temperature
without rigidity of the abdominal wall in a patient
previously well, except for some slight irregularity
of menstruation, seldom or never leave room for
doubt.

It may be impossible clinically to distinguish
rupture of an ectopic pregnancy from *severe
hæmorrhage from a Graafian follicle.* The latter
is a very rare occurrence and usually unaccompanied by any of the signs of pregnancy. In
a case seen by the author the palpitation, rapid
pulse, and nervous condition of the patient were
by one observer attributed to cardiac weakness
and hysteria. The low blood-pressure as shown
by the sphygmomanometer exposed the truly
critical condition of the patient.

(3) Symptoms in Cases with Subacute Hæmorrhage.

We must now consider diagnosis after repeated
bleedings have caused a hæmatocele to form.

Many cases come for diagnosis a short while after
an acute rupture of the sac, *or after repeated slight
hæmorrhages have led to the formation of a hæmatocele.*
At the time of observation the bleeding may have
stopped and the patient may have recovered
sufficiently to get about again. The previous
serious symptoms may have been attributed by the
patient to a simple fainting fit, or the doctor may
have thought the trouble due to a cardiac attack.

This mistake could only arise in those patients who have had moderate internal hæmorrhage, for in the extreme degrees the grave nature of the case cannot be missed.

After a moderate hæmorrhage the slight collapse is quickly recovered from, the pulse may become normal, and the temperature from subnormal may

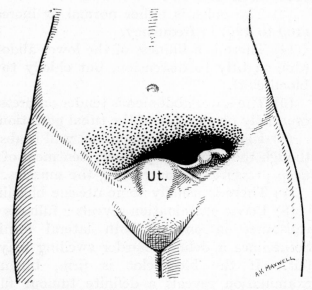

Fig. 35.—Diagram of a hæmatocele (from the front). (The black area indicates firm and older clot, the dotted portion represents looser and more recent clot.)

become slightly febrile. When there have been repeated slight hæmorrhages there may be no history of acute collapse, but usually with repeated attacks of pain the patient will have felt faint. Such a patient comes for advice either for abdominal pain and weakness, or for pain and uterine hæmorrhage. Occasionally retention of urine may cause advice to be sought.

Diagnosis is made by considering the history of repeated attacks of hypogastric or iliac pain, the irregularity in menstruation, and the conditions found on examination, which are as follows :

(1) The patient looks anæmic.

(2) The temperature is normal or febrile (100° F. or 101° F.).

(3) The pulse is either normal or increased (100 to 120) in frequency.

(4) There is a fullness of the lower abdomen (due slightly to distension, but chiefly to the blood-clot).

(5) The lower abdomen is tender on pressure, especially on the side of the tubal gestation.

(6) Rigidity of the abdominal wall is absent, though the patient may show resentment of any deep pressure by contracting the muscles.

(7) There is usually some uterine bleeding.

(8) Pelvic examination reveals a fullness and resistance in one or both lateral fornices. Sometimes a definite harder swelling may be felt. If the blood-clot is firm, bimanual examination reveals a definite tumour filling the pouch of Douglas. Pain is always elicited on pressure on the swelling (whether vaginally or per abdomen).

(9) There may be retention of urine or frequency of urination.

(10) On two occasions I have obtained a positive obturator or thigh-rotation test (see Chapter III).

Additional evidence of internal hæmorrhage may sometimes be obtained in the form of a bluish or

purplish discoloration in the region of the navel
(Cullen's sign).   Such discoloration, however, is
very inconstant.

Vomiting sometimes occurs with the attacks of
abdominal pain, but is not a constant nor import-

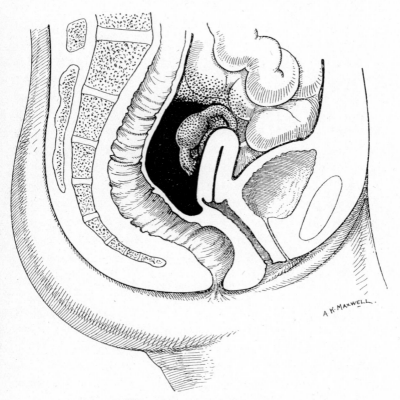

FIG. 36 —Diagram of a hæmatocele (lateral view).

ant feature.   Constipation may be present.   Diagnosis is usually clear from the above symptoms and
signs.   When the pregnancy has advanced two or
three months the softening of the cervix and enlargement of the breast may help in diagnosis (Fig. 36).

Differential diagnosis is sometimes difficult from pelvic **appendicitis, pyosalpinx,** or **retroverted gravid uterus.**

Pelvic appendicitis may give rise to nearly all the signs and symptoms of a small pelvic hæmatocele, and the two conditions are frequently confused in diagnosis. Hypogastric pain, vomiting, local tenderness, slight fever and tenderness on rectal or vaginal examination are commonly present in both conditions. Even the thigh-rotation test may be positive in both cases, and in neither instance should one expect to find abdominal-wall rigidity. The main points of distinction are that in an ectopic pregnancy there is nearly always *some* irregularity of menstruation or even definite amenorrhœa for a month or two, usually uterine bleeding, possibly the symptoms of early pregnancy and the appearance of anæmia, and the history of onset is suggestive of internal hæmorrhage and quite different from the usual onset of appendicitis in which the symptom-sequence may be definitely helpful in diagnosis.

With a *pyosalpinx* there should not be menstrual irregularity, though menorrhagia is not infrequent, and there should be a history of previous pelvic inflammation or of leucorrhœa, endometritis, or definite gonorrhœal infection. The uterine cervix will not be softened in pyosalpinx, and pain on micturition and retention of urine are less likely to occur.

A retroverted gravid uterus might be confused with an ectopic pregnancy which had gone on to the third or fourth month of gestation. Both may cause retention of urine. But if the bladder be emptied by catheter it should be possible to make out the determining factor in diagnosis, i.e. the absence or presence of the uterine fundus from the normal position. The bleeding from a retroverted gravid uterus would be that of fresh blood indicating threatening abortion, the blood lost in an ectopic gestation would usually be darker. Anæmia would only be observed in the ectopic pregnancy.

If the fœtus of an ectopic pregnancy survive the rupture until the later months of gestation, the condition will cause the formation of an abdominal tumour in which the fœtal parts may be felt easily under the abdominal wall, while at the same time the symptoms of pregnancy will be very evident. It is possible that acute symptoms might occur at this stage, but this is rare and need not be considered here.

CHAPTER XIII

CHOLECYSTITIS AND OTHER CAUSES OF ACUTE PAIN IN THE RIGHT UPPER QUADRANT OF THE ABDOMEN

SEVERE pain arising in, or chiefly localized to, the right hypochondriac region is usually due to one of the following conditions :

> Cholecystitis.
> Biliary colic.
> Inflamed or leaking duodenal ulcer.
> Rupture of gall-bladder or a biliary duct.
> Hepatitis.

But one always needs carefully to exclude

> Appendicitis.
> Renal pain or colic.
> Pleurisy or pleuro-pneumonia.

The gall-bladder and cystic duct may be regarded as a vermiform muscular tube which has a dilated extremity and opens mediately through the common bile-duct into the duodenum. In certain respects, therefore, it is analogous to the cæcal appendix. Further, it is common for a stone to stop up the cystic duct just as a concretion may occlude the lumen of the appendix. The chief difference between the two structures lies in the fact that fæcal material is common in the cæcal appendix

194

but never seen in the gall-bladder, though the *bacillus coli communis* (*Escherichia coli*) is frequently found in the latter.

Cholecystitis, or inflammation of the gall-bladder, may occur with or without the presence of gall-stones. Infection may gain access either from the blood-stream (more commonly) or from the intestine via the biliary ducts. The intensity of the inflammation varies greatly. Sometimes there is a mere catarrh of the mucous membrane lining the gall-bladder, which may be full of clear or bile-stained mucus, while frequently the inflammation involves the whole thickness of the bladder-wall, which becomes œdematous and friable. In extreme cases gangrene of part or the whole of the gall-bladder may occur. The inflamed viscus may have omentum adherent to it, but this does not occur quite so frequently as with an inflamed appendix. Rarely both gall-bladder and vermiform appendix may be simultaneously inflamed.

The contents of an inflamed gall-bladder consist either of clear or bile-stained mucus, or of muco-purulent bilious material sometimes containing much cholesterin in suspension, or accompanied by gall-stones. When gall-stones are present they may belong to any of the different varieties—the large barrel-shaped stone, the multiple small facetted stones, or the innumerable black pigment-calculi like small jet beads, which are sometimes embedded in a tar-like matrix.

When a gall-bladder is inflamed the overlying liver substance sometimes enlarges and projects downwards from the liver margin, forming one variety of Riedl's lobe.

The symptoms of cholecystitis are :
Pain.
Vomiting.
Fever.
Constipation.
Local tenderness in right hypochondrium.
Swelling in region of gall-bladder (sometimes).
Rigidity of overlying muscle (sometimes).
Jaundice (rarely).

The *pain* of cholecystitis varies according to whether or not there is a stone attempting to pass along the cystic duct. When there is no stone the pain is generally localized to the region of the gall-bladder, or if there be contiguous peritonitis (as is not infrequently the case) the pain may be diffused over the right hypochondriac region and even felt on top of the right shoulder. If the liver and gall-bladder are much enlarged downwards the pain may extend down almost to the iliac fossa.

When there is a stone in the neck of the gall-bladder or in the cystic duct the pain radiates also to the area beneath the inferior angle of the right scapula. This corresponds to the level of distribution of the eighth dorsal segment from which the gall-bladder derives its main nerve-supply. In uncomplicated cases pain is not felt in the right acromial or clavicular regions.

Vomiting is also a variable feature. It is slight in severity when there are no gall-stones and no peritonitis, but when either or both of these are present there may be constant vomiting or continual retching and bringing up of bilious material.

Local tenderness over the gall-bladder is a constant feature, and frequently when there is no muscular rigidity one can feel the rounded fundus of the viscus projecting below the inferior margin of the liver.   Usually the swelling is small, but occasionally it may be of considerable size and bulge down well into the right iliac fossa or into the umbilical region.

When the inflammation has spread to the parts around the gall-bladder there is usually rigidity of the right upper quadrant of the abdominal parietes, which thus protects the inflamed area.   In some cases of cholecystitis, however, there is no rigidity.

Fever is not usually high, but varies from 100° to 103° F. according to the extent of the inflammatory process and the virulence of the infection.   If the bile-ducts are simultaneously infected it is common to get higher and more irregular fever, occasional rigors, and in general more serious symptoms.

Constipation is usual, and is more obstinate if there be local peritonitis affecting the neighbouring coils of intestine.

The *pulse* is not of much diagnostic value.   It may remain steady and slow in spite of acute inflammation of the gall-bladder, the presence of biliary calculi, or even local peritonitis.   A rapid pulse in cholecystitis may be indicative of severe toxæmia, either from extending peritonitis or merely from toxic substances absorbed from the bile-ducts and gall-bladder.

Jaundice is not usual in cases of simple cholecystitis, nor is it the rule even when gall-stones are present, but there is frequently a history of jaundice occurring after previous attacks of acute abdominal pain.   This would suggest the previous passing of a gall-stone.

Differential diagnosis.—*Cholecystitis* is most commonly mistaken for *appendicitis*, or an *inflamed duodenal ulcer*.

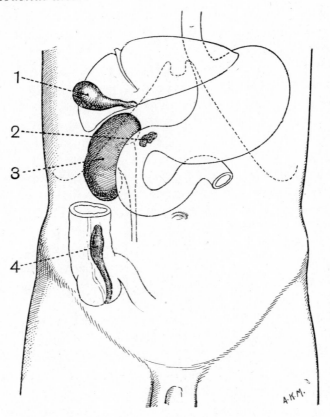

FIG. 37.—Diagram to illustrate the differential diagnosis of conditions simulating cholecystitis: (1) inflamed gall-bladder; (2) duodenal ulcer (with periduodenitis); (3) right kidney (with pyelitis); (4) inflamed ascending appendix.

The symptoms—pain, vomiting, constipation, fever, leucocytosis—are very similar to those of **appendicitis,** but the site of localized pain is in the one case in the right hypochondrium and in the other in the right lumbar or iliac regions. If any swelling be palpable its continuity with or distinction from the liver is of prime importance in diagnosis. It must be allowed that there are some cases, especially in fat subjects with a rather low-lying inflamed gall-bladder accompanied by local peritonitis and rigidity, in which a definite differentiation from appendicitis with local abscess is almost impossible before operation. A previous history of jaundice or biliary colic may be of assistance, or an account given of previous attacks suggestive of appendicitis might point to that disease. It must not be forgotten that it is not unknown for the two diseases to occur simultaneously.

Inflamed duodenal ulcer.—In the case of a duodenal ulcer which is threatening to perforate and has caused periduodenitis the local findings may be similar to those of cholecystitis with local peritonitis, but a careful inquiry into the *history* will distinguish. The pain which comes on about two and a half hours after meals and is relieved by taking food, the bringing up of " water-brash " and acid eructations, the attacks of flatulence, and possibly the occurrence of melæna may give a clear picture of ulcer. If time permits, the diagnosis of ulcer may be confirmed by noting deformity of the duodenal cap and a rapid emptying of the stomach as observed by X-rays after administration of a barium meal.

Retroperitoneal perforation of a duodenal ulcer may be attended by severe collapse at the onset, but the condition quickly localizes and leads to tenderness and swelling in the right loin. The perinephric tissues become œdematous, and there may be frequency of micturition and even hæmaturia from the irritation of the renal pelvis. There is great pain on pressure at the erector-costal angle. The diagnosis is difficult, since a primary renal condition is likely to be suspected.

Biliary colic (unassociated with inflammation of the gall-bladder) is distinguished from cholecystitis by its more acute onset, more paroxysmal and agonizing pain, and by the greater accompanying collapse. The abdominal wall over the gall-bladder is soft and yielding, though there may be local deep tenderness. The pain is usually radiating, being felt specially in the right subscapular area. It may also be felt on the left side, in which case there may be a complaint of a sense of constriction round the waist. This feeling of constriction, when present, is very characteristic of biliary colic. A subnormal temperature is more common than fever, and transient jaundice is common after the attack.

With **rupture of the gall-bladder** or of one of the bile-ducts there are usually the history and symptoms suggestive of biliary colic or cholecystitis, with a gradual extension of the painful area downwards until the whole abdomen is tender ; distension of the intestines increases and there is tenderness on rectal examination. Free fluid may sometimes be demonstrated. There is often a history of acute onset, with a subsequent remission of symptoms for a day or two and a final exacerbation of symptoms as the peritonitis spreads over the abdomen.

With retroperitoneal rupture of the bile-duct the symptoms and signs remain localized to the right side of the abdomen, and there is sometimes an irritation of the renal pelvis, causing pain on or frequency of micturition. This rare condition is, however, almost impossible to distinguish from cholecystitis or appendicitis before operation.

In **hepatitis** the tenderness is all over the liver, including *the lateral aspect* as ascertained by pressure in the lower intercostal spaces laterally, as well as in the right hypochondrium. This sign serves for diagnosis except in those cases where hepatitis coexists with the cholecystitis.

In **right basal pleuro-pneumonia or diaphragmatic pleurisy** fever is usually higher (104° or 105° F.), there may be an initial rigor, the right hypochondriac tenderness is more superficial, and by gradual coaxing the fingers may be pressed well into the subhepatic region, and there should be signs—at any rate fine crepitations—at the base of the right lung and pleura. Pain on top of the right shoulder would be much more likely to be met with in diaphragmatic pleurisy than in cholecystitis. The occurrence of hæmoptysis in any doubtful case would suggest either pneumonia or pulmonary infarct.

CHAPTER XIV

THE COLICS

TRUE abdominal colic is always caused by the violent peristaltic contraction of one of the involuntary muscular tubes, whose normal peristalsis is quite painless. The violence of the contraction is usually produced in an effort to overcome some obstacle which prevents the passage of the normal excretion or secretion. The pain is due to the stretching or distension of the tube, and the agony produced may be as severe as any to which a human being can be subjected.

The involuntary muscular tubes which may thus cause colic are :

> The stomach.
> Intestines.
> Cystic, hepatic, and common bile-ducts.
> The ureters.
> The uterus (and Fallopian tube).
> The pancreatic duct.

The main feature of severe colic is the occurrence of acute agonizing spasmodic pain, which doubles up the patient. It is associated in varying degree with the symptoms consequent on shock due to excessive stimulation of the sympathetic nervous system, e.g. pallor or lividity, weak pulse, vomiting, subnormal temperature or coldness of the body-surface. The pain is referred partly to the local site of origin, and partly to the area of nerve distribution of the segment of the spinal cord with

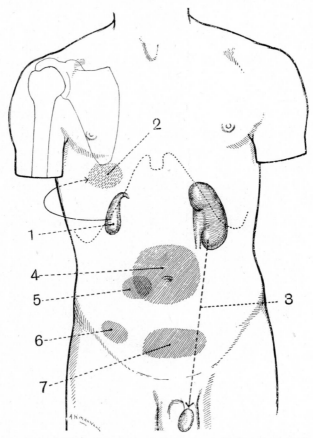

Fig. 38.—Diagram to show common sites to which pain is referred in the various forms of colic: (1) hypochondriac (over gall-bladder); (2) subscapular, painful areas in biliary colic; (3) renal colic; (4) small-gut pain and sometimes appendicular colic; (5) appendicular colic; (6) sensitive area in iliac abscess; (7) large-bowel pain. (See also Fig. 3 on page 11.)

which the affected part is associated. The abdominal muscles, in common with many other of the voluntary muscles, may remain contracted and rigid during the height of the pain, but they relax when the spasm of pain subsides, and the fingers may then be pressed fairly easily into the abdominal cavity, though there may be local tenderness over the affected viscus.

In the general diagnosis of a colic the following points may help :

(1) In colic the patient is usually very restless, and flings himself about as if to find some relief from the pain which grips him. A flexed position of the body may be adopted during the pain.

(2) In colic pressure to the abdomen sometimes relieves the pain—an occurrence not usual in other acute conditions.

(3) The pain usually comes in paroxysms lasting a variable time.

(4) Though occasionally rigid during the paroxysms the abdominal wall is soft between the bouts of pain. In sudden acute peritonitis it remains rigid all the time.

(5) In many of the colics the pain-distribution is almost diagnostic. (Fig. 38.)

Intestinal colic.—*Colic of the small intestine* is sometimes caused by catarrhal enteritis due to the irritation of improper food, ptomaine poisoning, or the toxins of some fevers. It is met with in more severe degree in that rare condition termed " enterospasm," and in cases of organic obstruction to the small intestine. The pain is acute and griping, is referred to the epigastric or umbilical region, and is accompanied sometimes by local areas of distension where gurgling sounds may be heard, and sometimes felt by the palpating hand. Vomiting may take place, and peristalsis may occasionally be seen through the abdominal wall. When due to enteritis the pain is generally soon followed by diarrhœa, the nature of which may give the clue to the cause of the pain. When due to organic obstruction the attacks will occur from time to time till a final attack of acute intestinal obstruction occurs. Enterospasm cannot well be distinguished from organic obstruction. When severe pain, assumed to be due to intestinal colic, persists for more than three or four hours, the condition is generally one needing surgical intervention.

Lead colic is a form of colic of the small intestine which is accompanied by constipation. The pain may be extreme and the collapse of the patient severe. During the spasms of pain the abdominal wall may be rigid. Other signs and symptoms pointing to lead poisoning (blue line on gums, severe constipation, local paralysis, etc.) may be present, and the patient's occupation is usually that of a painter, or one who comes in contact with paint.

Colic of the large intestine is very frequent, but the pain occasioned by the large bowel is seldom so acute or prostrating as that resulting from colic of the small bowel. The pain is referred chiefly to the hypogastrium. The causes are either severe constipation, due to hard scybalous masses, colitis or dysentery, or some form of stricture of the large bowel. Pain in the colon is often more accurately localized by the patient than is the pain of small-bowel colic.

Diagnosis.—In any case of intestinal colic diagnosis is greatly aided by the history, for the history of eating of tainted food or the knowledge that similar attacks have occurred in other members of the household, the occurrence of previous similar attacks in one who is a painter by trade, or an account given of former bouts of dysentery, may throw considerable light on the problem. By obtaining a careful history it should also be possible to exclude appendicular colic. The occurrence of diarrhœa would usually exclude intestinal obstruction, but it must be recollected that loose motions are sometimes seen with an intussusception (q.v.). Local or diffuse peritonitis must be excluded by noting the absence of rigidity when the severe pain subsides, the relief obtained by gentle pressure on the abdomen, and the absence of tenderness of the pelvic peritoneum.

If attacks of small-intestine colic recur from time to time and lead to loss of weight, the possibility of organic obstruction (by adhesions, bands, tuberculous stricture or neoplasm) must be considered, nor is it wise to delay too long before advising radiographic examination of the intestinal tract. Tuberculous mesenteric glands frequently lead to subacute attacks of intestinal colic, and in these cases a radiograph may show evidence of calcification of the glands.

Similarly when there are recurrent attacks of distension of the large bowel, accompanied by colic and constipation, it is wise to suspect carcinoma or stricture of the colon or rectum, and certainty on the question must be obtained by the proper diagnostic procedure (see Chapter IX).

Biliary colic is caused by the passing of a stone or inspissated bile through the cystic, hepatic, or common bile-ducts. It varies considerably in intensity according to the difficulty which the stone experiences in traversing the ducts. The pain is usually sudden in onset and severe in intensity. Vomiting is common and collapse may be so severe that the observer may consider the patient *in extremis*. Occasionally death has actually occurred during an attack of biliary colic, and the writer has known one such case, but fortunately this event is exceedingly rare. Generally the patient writhes in agony, but in the worst cases may lie still with pinched, blue face, cold extremities, and weak pulse. The pain is felt :

(1) In the right hypochondrium, which is usually tender on pressure.

(2) Below the inferior angle of the right scapula.

(3) Occasionally at the same levels on the other side of the body.

(4) Infrequently it may be referred to the right acromial and lower cervical region.

The common position of the pain corresponds to the distribution of the nerves from the eighth and ninth dorsal segment of the spinal cord.

Jaundice is not a necessary accompaniment of biliary colic, but in slight degree it is a frequent sequel.

Diagnosis is usually fairly clear on account of the intensity and distribution of the pain and the absence of local abdominal rigidity when the pain passes off. *When rigidity persists* in the right hypochondrium there must be accompanying cholecystitis or *local peritonitis*. A leaking or inflamed duodenal ulcer causes also persistent rigidity, but in the case of ulcer there should be a definite history suggestive of that condition (see Chapter XIII).

Renal colic is caused by the passage of a small

stone, a portion of blood-clot or inspissated pus, oxalate crystals or uratic débris down the ureter, by the impaction of a stone in the renal pelvis, and sometimes by sudden kinking of the uretero-pelvic junction when there is an unduly mobile kidney. It is sometimes, but by no means always, accompanied by hæmaturia.

The symptoms are usually characteristic. The patient is seized with sudden pain starting in the loin and often radiating to the corresponding testicle or groin, or, (in women), to the vulva. In some cases there is extensive superficial hyperæsthesia of the abdominal wall either in front or posteriorly. In severe cases there is violent restlessness. Vomiting is common. There may be frequency of urination and pain on performing the act. Hæmaturia may accompany or follow the pain. Renal colic in males by no means always radiates to the testicle, and it must be remembered that pain due to inflammation of the appendix is sometimes felt in the testicle.

Diagnosis.—The distribution of the pain is characteristic, and local examination of the loin may reveal a tender and possibly enlarged kidney. An X-ray examination may show a stone to be present, but there are many cases of renal colic in which no stone is seen by the X-rays, yet a small stone is passed later. Minor degrees of ureteric colic are frequently misdiagnosed appendicular colic, especially when a radiograph is unsuccessful in revealing the small calculus.

Uterine colic.—*Dysmenorrhœa.*—The pain caused by the uterus in its attempt to expel either a fœtus, a polypus, a membranous cast, or even blood-clot may be very severe. The pain is referred chiefly to the lower lumbar region, but in severe cases it may radiate down the thighs and over the hips. Vomiting and retching may occur.

Spasmodic dysmenorrhœa may cause the patient to writhe. Since with any abdominal pain in women the menstrual history would be inquired into, and with spasmodic dysmenorrhœa vaginal and pelvic examination would show no special reason for pain of uterine origin (apart perhaps from a pin-hole os and small cervix), there should be little difficulty in diagnosis.

Gastric colic.—Attacks of severe epigastric pain of a colicky nature sometimes occur in those who are the subject of pyloric stenosis, due to ulcer or neoplasm. In such cases the peristaltic wave can often be seen going from left to right, and the out-line of the dilated stomach may readily be recognized through the abdominal wall. The pain is referred to the area of distribution of the tenth dorsal segment, chiefly on the left side.

Severe pain may also be caused by a sudden hæmorrhage taking place into the stomach. In such cases there is usually a history suggestive of gastric ulcer. The severe pain and collapse and epigastric tenderness may lead one to diagnose intestinal obstruction or gastric perforation. But the sudden anæmia and the vomiting of altered blood (which usually occurs) will give the clue to the correct diagnosis.

Pancreatic colic.—Very occasionally obstruction to the duct of Wirsung may give rise to colic. Severe pain, sometimes radiating to the left shoulder, may be felt, and there will be symptoms of pancreatic derangement, but the condition is probably rarely correctly diagnosed before operation.

CHAPTER XV

THE EARLY DIAGNOSIS OF ABDOMINAL INJURIES [1]

EVERY case of abdominal injury which is obviously of a serious nature is nowadays removed to the care of the surgeon ; but since there are many cases in which, though serious injury has resulted from the injury, the symptoms are not obvious and indeed may remain latent for some hours, it is useful to summarize the main points in diagnosis.

We shall confine ourselves to the consideration of those injuries in which there is no open wound of the parietes, for when a stab or penetrating wound of the abdominal wall exists there should be no question that the treatment is surgical.

Non-penetrating injuries of the abdomen are most commonly due to severe crushes, as would follow from a heavy vehicle running over the abdomen. Another type of violence is the sharp circumscribed blow due to a kick, punch, or the sudden impinging of any hard body against the abdominal wall. Severe injury may also follow the strain on the visceral attachments consequent on a fall from a height, or a sudden trip-up causing a violent fall forward. When violence is applied

[1] The author is indebted to the publishers of *The Dictionary of Practical Medicine* for permission to abstract from his article in that publication.

210

against the abdominal wall the kind of injury produced depends to a certain extent upon the preparedness of the patient for the blow and the consequent rigidity or flaccidity of the abdominal muscles. If the muscle is taken unawares more serious intra-abdominal mischief is to be expected, whereas if the muscle be rigid it may mitigate or prevent injury of the underlying viscera.

Any injury of the abdominal wall, however slight, may be accompanied by serious lesions of the viscera, and the latter may be seriously injured without any visible sign of injury to the abdominal wall. When there is no external wound the thought of visceral injury may not be present in the mind, and grave lesions may be allowed to progress considerably before they are noticed.

The solid viscera of the abdomen (liver, spleen, pancreas, kidneys) are situated high up in the abdomen largely under cover of the ribs ; the hollow tubes (intestines, bladder, ureter, and stomach) are more exposed to injury.

Injury to solid viscera causes hæmorrhage, injury to the hollow viscera usually causes peritonitis, whilst both types of lesion are accompanied by shock.

Shock is shown by pallor, feeble pulse, sweating, slow shallow respiration, and cold extremities, but unless there is some serious lesion the symptoms soon subside. If the state of shock lasts longer and seems out of proportion to the evidence of intra-abdominal injury, examination may reveal a pneumothorax or other chest-lesion. Injuries of the upper abdomen cause more serious shock than those of the hypogastric region. Renal contusions also cause severe shock. The observer should recollect that in a very shocked patient the reflexes are diminished and consequently rigidity of the abdominal wall may be absent even in the presence of peritoneal irritation (Bradford, B., *et al.*, *Annals of Surg.*, 1946, vol. 123, p. 32).

If the symptoms of shock do not pass off within six hours, hæmorrhage or peritonitis is almost certainly an additional factor.

Owing to the anatomical disposition of the parts **hæmorrhage** usually follows lesions of the upper zone in which lie the liver and spleen. The main abdominal vessels are more likely to be injured by violence directed against the central portion of the abdomen. When the liver or spleen is severely torn, the symptoms of shock and hæmorrhage are extreme, and death frequently follows soon after the injury. In lesser degrees of injury of the solid viscera (or of the mesenteric blood-vessels) evidences of bleeding gradually assert themselves. Increasing restlessness, and pain, progressive pallor of the lips and finger-nails, a rising pulse-rate, and the demonstration of movable dullness in the flanks are sufficiently indicative. Occasionally the symptoms of hæmorrhage may abate for a day or two, and then become alarmingly evident after some exertion, e.g. straining on the bed-pan. This is more likely to occur after injuries to the spleen. The pulse-rate is a good but by no means infallible guide in abdominal hæmorrhage. It may continue fairly slow (not above 100) till the abdomen is full of blood, and then suddenly bound up to a rapid rate. Presumably the increase in rate takes place when the cardio-vascular compensating mechanism fails.

Contusion or rupture of the kidney is frequently

accompanied by very severe and alarming shock, which generally passes off within an hour or two (cp. the " kidney-punch " in boxing). The later symptoms depend on the extent of the injury and the condition of the renal capsule. In slight cases where the capsule remains intact, hæmaturia, local tenderness, and sometimes renal colic due to the passage of clots down the ureter, comprise all the symptoms. If the renal capsule be torn a retro-peritoneal hæmatoma is formed, and sometimes urine is extravasated into the cellular tissues behind and around the kidney ; this leads to cellulitis accompanied by malaise, irregular fever, and local swelling, tenderness, and muscular resistance. An abscess may result. If the urine be infected the symptoms are more acute. Should the peritoneal covering of the kidney be torn, symptoms of intra-peritoneal hæmorrhage will result. Most cases of hæmaturia resulting from renal contusion stop spontaneously, but a rising pulse-rate, accompanied by continuing hæmaturia or by an increasing retro-peritoneal peri-renal swelling, calls urgently for exploration.

Peritonitis is usually consequent on rupture of the hollow viscera. The intestines, bladder, and stomach are most commonly injured, the gall-bladder and ureters rarely. Sometimes the injury is only sufficient to bruise the walls of the viscus. If the stomach be thus contused the result is vomiting and sometimes hæmatemesis ; if the colon be bruised the passage of blood per anum and diarrhœa due to traumatic colitis may follow.

Bruising of the bladder causes slight hæmaturia, but if the contusion be severe there may be vomiting and local muscular rigidity, even though no rupture has occurred.

Rupture of intestine [1] is the commonest cause of peritonitis after abdominal injury; it is a condition fraught with danger of almost certain death if not diagnosed early, yet the signs and symptoms are often equivocal for some hours. Generally the tear only involves a portion of the circumference of the gut, but occasionally a complete severance is caused and a gap left between the two ends which may be temporarily closed by contraction of the involuntary intestinal muscle. When intestine is injured its peristaltic movements stop owing to a reflex or direct paresis of its walls. If the rent be small the edges of the mucous membrane pout and fill the small gap; a small amount of intestinal contents escapes and sets up a local plastic peritonitis with deposit of lymph which glues together the coils of intestine. The patient takes nothing by the mouth, and the gut remains at rest. A lull in the symptoms gives a false security. After a few hours, when the observer may have decided that there is no serious intra-abdominal lesion, food is taken, the intestines are excited to peristaltic contraction and the opening in the gut is unsealed. Peritonitis then develops more or less rapidly according to the size of the opening and the number of adhesions.

The important earlier signs of peritonitis are:

    Pain.

    Local tenderness.

    Local muscular rigidity.

[1] *Vide* Cope, " The Early Diagnosis and Treatment of Ruptured Intestines," *Proceedings of Royal Society of Medicine*, 1914.

Vomiting.

Shallow abdominal respiration.

The later evidences of peritoneal infection are :

Elevation of pulse and temperature.

Increasing distension.

Tenderness of pelvic peritoneum.

Movable dullness in the flanks.

Obliteration or diminution of liver-dullness (caused by gas in front of the liver).

The patient often has an anxious facial expression and may show unusual restlessness. In injuries of the upper abdomen importance must be attached to the shifting of the pain to the hypogastrium, due to the inflammation caused by the escaped intestinal contents which gravitate to the pelvis. The absence of intestinal sounds on repeated auscultation of the abdomen would be in favour of some intestinal injury.

A plain X-ray photograph of the abdomen may be useful by showing free gas localized near a ruptured portion of gut.

The prognosis in cases of ruptured intestine is very bad, unless diagnosis is made and operation undertaken soon after the injury. Hence the need for early diagnosis.

Provided there be no lesion in the chest, and that renal trauma can be excluded, one is probably dealing with a case of ruptured intestine in the following conditions :

(1) When severe abdominal pain persists for more than about six hours after an injury, if the pain be accompanied by either (*a*) vomiting, especially bilious vomiting ; or (*b*) a pulse gradually

rising from the normal ; or (c) persistent local rigidity tending to extend ; or (d) deep local tenderness with shallow respiration.

(2) When abdominal pain is absent or very slight, and anæmia is not increasing, but the pulse rises steadily hour by hour, and the patient is very restless or listless.

When marked diminution of the liver-dullness occurs with any of the above symptoms, or if there be signs of free fluid in the abdomen or rectal examination shows the pelvic peritoneum to be very tender, the indications for operation would be imperative.

It is assumed that the opening of the abdomen would be advised without any delay if the symptoms of peritonitis were quite typical.

It is possible for the duodenum and parts of the colon to be ruptured behind the peritoneum. The symptoms are then due to a retro-peritoneal cellulitis, with some inflammation of the contiguous peritoneum, viz. local pain and muscular rigidity, shallow respiration, vomiting, rise of pulse-rate and of temperature. In a case of retroperitoneal injury to the duodenum which was under my care the pain at first was very slight but became greater hour by hour till I felt constrained to open the abdomen though there were few local signs to guide one. A very important diagnostic sign (when present) is surgical emphysema of the retroperitoneal tissues.

Rupture of the urinary bladder usually occurs in connexion with fractured pelvis, but may ersult from a blow on the hypogastrium when the viscus is distended. In children the bladder is situated higher up in the abdomen, and is therefore more liable to injury. The symptoms vary according as the rent is intra- or extra-peritoneal. If within the peritoneal cavity, symptoms of peritonitis ensue, but it must be remembered that sterile urine does not at first cause a very acute inflammatory reaction. There may be hæmaturia.

Rupture outside the peritoneum tends to extravasation of urine and consequent cellulitis in the suprapubic and perineal regions.

In a child with fractured pelvis the membranous urethra may be torn completely across, and the neck of the bladder with the torn portion of attached urethra may retract from the triangular ligament. In such cases the bladder-sphincter may remain contracted and the viscus become over-distended. A tense and tender swelling will thus be detectable in the hypogastrium. The tenseness and tenderness of the lower abdomen thus produced may cause the diagnosis of peritonitis to be made erroneously.

RUPTURE OF THE STOMACH quickly leads to symptoms of general peritonitis ; it is generally accompanied by some other lesion such as injury to the spleen or liver. The part of the stomach likely to be ruptured by injury is that part which is seldom the site of ruptured ulcer, i.e. the greater curvature. The gas which escapes may for a time be localized and form an area of superficial tympanitic resonance on percussion.

The pancreas is rarely injured, and the symptoms of such injury are in no way distinctive. Shock is always great.

Diagnosis of abdominal injuries.—The essential point in diagnosis is to estimate the different proportions which shock, hæmorrhage, and peritonitis take in the production of the observed symptoms, and to judge from this the viscus injured and the nature of the lesion.

It is frequently impossible to give a definite opinion for a few hours after the accident. Initial shock usually subsides within two or three hours, and then symptoms of hæmorrhage or peritonitis become increasingly evident. If shock is still present after three hours there is nearly always some serious visceral lesion. Pain, vomiting, local or general muscular rigidity, tenderness, alteration of pulse-rate, shallow respiration, diminution of liver-dullness, free fluid in the abdomen—these are the main symptoms to note. By taking into consideration the part of the abdomen struck, it is possible in many cases to say which viscus is injured and what is the nature of the injury.

In cases of suspected rupture of the bladder two additional means of diagnosis are available :

(1) The bladder is emptied by a catheter and a measured quantity of boric acid or saline solution is introduced and again drawn off. Any serious discrepancy between the amount put in and drawn out suggests rupture of the bladder.

(2) Cystoscopy may show a rent in the bladder, but this should only be carried out by an expert in the use of the cystoscope.

Differential diagnosis.—It is very important always to *examine the thorax carefully* for pneumothorax or hæmopneumothorax. Symptoms very suggestive of serious abdominal injury may be produced by either of these lesions. Abdominal pain and rigidity and the general signs of shock and hæmorrhage may follow a fracture of rib with rupture of lung and consequent presence of blood and air in the pleural cavity. Hence the need of careful thoracic examination. In cases of doubt radiography of the chest, by means of a portable X-ray apparatus, would clearly show whether there were a pneumothorax.

CHAPTER XVI

THE ACUTE ABDOMEN IN THE TROPICS [1]

In tropical climes there are several common acute abdominal conditions which are seldom seen in temperate regions. For the most part these are the manifestations of malaria and dysentery. Some of the most common are:

Hepatitis (amœbic or malarial).
Acute liver-abscess.
Rupture of liver-abscess.
Dysenteric typhlitis.
Acute or subacute dysenteric perforation.
Perforation of a typhoidal ulcer.

Pain in the right upper quadrant of the abdomen which in temperate climes usually indicates cholecystitis or duodenal ulcer, in the tropics frequently means either amœbic or malarial hepatitis.

AMŒBIC HEPATITIS

It is essential for the practitioner in the tropics to have a sound knowledge of the symptoms of amœbic hepatitis, since it is the first stage toward amœbic abscess of the liver, and prompt and early recognition and treatment of the hepatitis will save

[1] See *The Surgical Aspects of Dysentery*, by Zachary Cope (Henry Frowde and Hodder & Stoughton).

many a patient from the inconvenience and danger of surgical interference.

Hepatitis may develop during the course of an acute amœbic colitis, or it may come on at a period remote from the dysenteric attack. The amœbæ travel to the liver via the radicles of the portal vein, and lodging in the portal capillaries cause extensive inflammation.

Symptoms.—There are five constant features and many inconstant symptoms to be looked for in amœbic hepatitis. The constant features are :

(1) Enlargement of the liver.
(2) Pain and tenderness in the hepatic region.
(3) Fever.
(4) Leucocytosis.
(5) Reaction to emetine.

The common though inconstant features are :

History of dysentery.
Jaundice.
Pain in the right shoulder-region, or in iliac region.
A rigor.
Lassitude and malaise.
Foul tongue.
Sweating.

The occurrence of fever, with an enlarged painful liver, in a person who is or has been living in a tropical country should always lead one to suspect amœbic hepatitis, whether there is a definite history or not of amœbic dysentery. The occurrence of leucocytosis (15,000 to 20,000) is corroborative evidence. The presence of any of the inconstant symptoms may be taken as confirmation. The diagnosis is always clinched by the rapid, often dramatically rapid, subsidence of symptoms under treatment by hypodermic injection of emetine hydrochloride one grain daily for ten days. The symptoms begin to abate after the administration of two or three doses.

Differential diagnosis.—There are several pitfalls that lie in wait for the unwary. *Malaria* may cause a hepatitis with jaundice. This can be excluded by examining the blood for the malarial parasite. Cholecystitis may be wrongly diagnosed because the pain may be most evident in the gallbladder region. If the pain be also referred to the right iliac region, there is a simulation of appendicitis. *In a tropical country it would be a wise procedure for the surgeon to try the effect of a short course of emetine before operating on any but the most fulminating types of appendicitis and cholecystitis.*

Acute pain in the right lower quadrant of the abdomen when occurring in a patient residing in a temperate clime is usually due to appendicitis. In the tropics, however, one must also consider (in addition to hepatitis) :

> Dysenteric typhlitis.
> Cæcal perforation with local abscess.
> Leaking hepatic abscess.

The insidious nature of amœbic colitis permits considerable pathological lesions to exist without many symptoms. Ulceration in the cæcum is frequently accompanied by considerable swelling of the gut, but may be unaccompanied by any dysenteric symptoms—on the contrary, constipation may be the complaint. If then, in such a case, pain is suddenly complained of in the right iliac fossa, the temperature becomes elevated and vomiting occurs, and on examination a tender lump is found in the appendicular region, the conditions for a false diagnosis are evident. The surgeon practising in the tropics must not be too ready to operate on painful swellings in the right iliac fossa. The examination of the fæces for amœbæ, and the trial of treatment by emetine for two or three days, are useful and often necessary preliminary procedures, for operation on cases of amœbic typhlitis is fraught with peril.

Perforation of the cæcum may take place insidiously, and adhesions may limit infection to the iliac fossa. Such cases, apart from the history, are almost indistinguishable from those of appendicular abscess.

Since local abscess will always need to be opened, the actual mistake as to the cause of the abscess makes little difference save that more rapid healing will ensue if emetine is simultaneously given in cases of amœbic dysentery.

Simulation of appendicitis by a leaking hepatic abscess is a rare event, but an instance has come under my observation.

General abdominal pain may be produced in the tropics by the usual causes described in the different chapters of this book, but in addition one may have to deal with :

Rupture of liver-abscess into the general
peritoneal cavity.

Rupture of dysenteric ulcer.

Rupture of typhoidal ulcer.

Cholera sicca.

Ruptured spleen.

Rupture of liver-abscess into the general peritoneal
cavity is not common, but is sufficiently frequent
to bear in mind as a possible cause of the acute
abdomen. It would give rise to all the symptoms
of diffuse peritonitis (q.v.), and unless the patient
was known to have been suffering from recent
liver disease it is unlikely that the proper diagnosis
would be made before the abdomen was opened.

Rupture of dysenteric ulcer into peritoneal cavity.
—The most common sites for perforation are the
cæcum and sigmoid colon. Consideration of the
grades of acuteness of the amœbic ulceration will
explain partly the difference of symptoms which
may result after perforation. In the acute type of
inflammation, in which masses of the mucous membrane are cast off as gangrenous sloughs, there is
little reaction in the bowel wall, and ulceration
may penetrate through to the peritoneal coat before
time has been allowed for protective adhesions to
form. In such cases, when the bowel finally gives
way, the peritoneal cavity may suddenly be flooded
with fæcal material and fatal general peritonitis
rapidly ensue.

If, however, the ulcer is subacute and the wall of
the colon only permits a gradual erosion, there may
be time for omentum or intestine to adhere to the
peritoneum covering the base of the ulcer. Ad-

hesions may therefore prevent the rupture, or may surround the diseased area so that, when rupture takes place, the escape of gut-contents is into a limited space.   A localized abscess then results.

There is an intermediate type of lesion in which perforation may not occur, but an escape of organisms may take place through the thinned ulcer-base into the peritoneal cavity, though there is no general escape of intestinal contents, and the base of the perforating ulcer is very soon sealed up by adhesions.

The *symptoms* produced by perforation in a case of dysentery will vary in severity according to pathological type.

(*a*) If fæcal flooding of the general peritoneal cavity occurs, the symptoms indicating the catastrophe will be an onset or increase of abdominal pain, vomiting, collapse, rising pulse-rate, distension, and abdominal-wall rigidity.   In patients who are exhausted by the dysenteric condition, and in whom abdominal pain and distension have been considerable, rigidity may not be a marked feature, and the exacerbation of symptoms may not easily be distinguished from the collapse of severe toxæmia.

(*b*) If the leakage is gradual, and adhesions occur, the signs of local abscess will develop.

(*c*) In the intermediate type the symptoms will be those of subacute peritonitis.

Rupture of a typhoid ulcer may occur in some cases of ambulatory typhoid fever, so that a person previously supposed to be in fair health may be brought in with symptoms of peritonitis of recent origin.   The symptoms would at first be more evident in the lower abdomen, since it is usually in the ileum that the perforation occurs.   Unless there were a history suggestive of the onset of typhoid fever it is unlikely that the condition would be distinguished from appendicitis with pelvic peritonitis.

Rupture of spleen.—In tropical and subtropical countries where malaria is endemic there are many of the population who have enlarged spleens. Slight trauma may occasionally cause rupture of such an enlarged spleen, and very rarely rupture may occur spontaneously.

The symptoms would be collapse and the signs of internal hæmorrhage. The only hope of cure would be by operation to remove the spleen.

Cholera sicca.—There are some cases of cholera in which the patient is seized with violent abdominal pains and symptoms of very severe toxæmia, which may cause death before the stools have become frequent and characteristic. Such an acute condition might possibly simulate other forms of the acute abdomen, but the absence of abdominal rigidity and the severity of the toxæmia would put one on guard, and the prevalence of cholera would make one suspect the true cause. Moreover, in cholera sicca there is no rallying from the initial collapse. If the patient live long enough the characteristic stools would appear and clinch the diagnosis.

Heat-stroke.—In very hot seasons and in places where a number of heat-strokes are occurring it is well to remember that the initial stage of some cases of heat-stroke may show gastro-intestinal symptoms. It is very seldom, however, that there could be any mistaking these symptoms for an acute abdominal disease, for there are always other symptoms—dry skin, hyperpyrexia, mental dullness, etc.—which would guide one correctly.

Abdominal symptoms due to salt deficiency.—In tropical climes, as a result of the great heat and consequent excessive sweating, there may result a state of salt deficiency. This may give rise to severe cramps which may affect the muscles of the abdominal wall and cause such great pain, collapse, rigidity, and tenderness that the observer may even diagnose the condition as one due to perforation of a peptic ulcer. A quick test of the chlorides in the urine should be made and if there be serious deficiency salt should be administered promptly. If the condition be due to deficiency of salt the symptoms then soon subside (Stening, M. J. L., 1945. *Journ. of Royal Nav. Med. Serv.*, vol. 31, p. 129).

CHAPTER XVII

ACUTE ABDOMINAL DISEASE WITH GENITO-URINARY SYMPTOMS

ACUTE abdominal disease with genito-urinary symptoms may be due to primary disease of the genito-urinary organs, or to secondary irritation of those organs consequent on disease of other viscera. The main symptoms which may call attention are :

(1) Painful swelling in the position of the kidney.

(2) Renal colic.

(3) Disorders of micturition—pain, frequency, retention.

(4) Abnormalities of urine—hæmaturia, albuminuria.

(5) Pain in testicle or along spermatic cord.

(6) Tenderness at the right erector-costal angle.

(1) A *pyonephrosis* or a *hydronephrosis* may give rise to acute symptoms. In each case there will be found a rounded tender swelling in the loin. The tumour will be felt to fill out the posterior lumbar region. The colon may be felt to the front and inner aspect of the swelling, but if the loin is well filled by the tumour that alone is usually quite sufficient to diagnose a renal swelling. In both pyonephrosis and hydronephrosis there should be a history of previous urinary trouble. Acute attacks of pain are prone to occur in a recurring

hydronephrosis, and gastro-intestinal symptoms (flatulence and vomiting) may accompany the attacks. If seen during an attack, however, the swelling is characteristic. In a pyonephrosis there are usually the signs of toxic absorption—fever, furred tongue, and a toxæmic appearance. With a hydronephrosis the symptoms are less severe. Sometimes it is difficult to obtain a history of renal symptoms, and then it may be impossible by clinical examination alone to diagnose a pyonephrosis with accompanying perinephritis from other causes of local suppuration, such as appendicitis or diverticulitis—particularly in a fat patient.

Polycystic disease of the kidneys may give rise to uræmia with vomiting and abdominal distension. This might be mistaken for intestinal obstruction, but the presence of tumours in both loins would make one suspicious, and the occurrence of albuminuria and high blood-pressure would make the diagnosis almost certain. A polycystic kidney usually has an irregular surface due to the smooth cysts which vary considerably in size.

(2) Pain of the type of *renal colic* may be caused by:
    Stone in pelvis of kidney.
    Stone in ureter.
    Blood-clot or uratic débris in ureter.
    Dietl's crisis.
    Appendicitis.

In renal colic the pain starts in the loin and frequently radiates to the groin or to the corresponding testicle. It may be due to anything solid or semi-solid passing down the ureter, or to a sudden kink in the ureter due to a movable kidney (Dietl's crisis).

There is usually no difficulty in diagnosis, though occasionally appendicular colic or even appendicitis may cause pain of a similar nature. But in appendicitis severe enough to cause the simulation of renal colic there will usually be persistent local muscular rigidity, which is not usually found in renal colic. (See Chapter XIV.)

(3) *Pain on or frequency of urination* is found in nearly all cases of pyelitis, and in many cases of renal colic, but it is often also noted in appendicitis and other causes of pelvic peritonitis. Examination of the urine will prove or disprove a pyelitis.

In appendicitis pain on, or a frequency of, urination may be due to irritation of the renal pelvis, ureter, or bladder by the inflamed appendix or contiguous peritonitis. When this symptom is accompanied by pelvic tenderness, or a tender lump felt per rectum, or a positive obturator-test, the appendix will usually be found in the pelvis irritating the bladder. When unaccompanied by the other signs the appendix is generally either near the kidney or at the pelvic brim.

In pelvic hæmatocele due to a ruptured ectopic gestation there are frequently urinary symptoms. Sometimes there is retention of urine, sometimes slight pain or frequency. In a very anæmic woman with abdominal pain and urinary symptoms it is well to think of ectopic gestation. Acute distension of the bladder may cause very severe hypogastric pain and sometimes pain in the lower lumbar region ; there should be no difficulty in palpating or percussing out the distended bladder, and one must not be misled by the fact that urine may be passed by the process of overflow incontinence. In those rarer cases in which the bladder does not distend upwards but rather backwards and upwards it may be difficult to make out its position by percussion, but bimanual examination will determine it.

(4) *Hæmaturia* frequently follows renal colic, and may sometimes enable one to trace to its source a renal pain that was not quite typical.

Albuminuria is an exceedingly important symptom, for uræmic symptoms may very closely simulate intestinal obstruction, and it may only be by the discovery of albuminuria that one is put on the right track. Many patients with nephritis have undergone needless and harmful abdominal section because of neglect to test the urine. Toxic albuminuria is found in many septic states of the abdomen, but it is usually not difficult to judge when the toxæmia is severe enough to produce that symptom.

(5) *Pain in the testicle* is met with in renal colic and in a few cases of appendicitis. In the latter instance it may either be due to irritation of the sympathetic branch which accompanies the spermatic artery, or be a true referred segmental pain across the tenth spinal segment.

Torsion of the imperfectly descended testicle may cause extreme pain in the inguinal region. Vomiting occurs and shock may be severe. The pain has the usual sickening character of testicular pain. The absence of the testicle from the same side of the scrotum will be noted and make diagnosis easy.

Thrombosis or suppurative phlebitis of the veins of the spermatic cord causes pain in the inguinal region and sometimes the iliac region of the abdomen. But the swelling and painful area extend right down to the testicle, which becomes swollen and painful.

Retraction of the testicle is occasionally noted in cases of appendicitis.   It is due to reflex contraction of the cremaster muscle.

(6) *Tenderness* on pressure *at the* right *erector-costal angle* (i.e. the usual position for eliciting tenderness of the right kidney) is noted in many cases of appendicitis, especially when the appendix is retrocæcal in position.

Renal symptoms may be caused by any retro-peritoneal lesion in the region of the renal pelvis ; thus a duodenal ulcer leaking posteriorly or a retro-peritoneal perforation of the common bile-duct may cause frequency of micturition or even slight hæmaturia.

CHAPTER XVIII

THE DIAGNOSIS OF ACUTE PERITONITIS

APART from hæmorrhage, the cause of death in nearly all fatal acute abdominal cases is either secondary peritonitis or acute paralytic or mechanical obstruction of the intestines. Spreading or general peritonitis, with consequent toxæmia and secondary shock, is the commonest single cause of death. Most cases, unless the patient is actually moribund, sooner or later demand an opening of the abdomen for drainage purposes. At operation fluid may easily be obtained for examination, but even before operation it is possible to obtain some by puncturing the abdomen in the midline midway between the navel and the pubis by means of a fine bore needle. The exudate is stained for organisms and examined microscopically. By noting the number and type of leucocytes and the amount of phagocytosis one may estimate the patient's resistance.

Infective organisms may reach the peritoneum :

(1) Through a wound of the abdominal wall.
(2) Via the blood-stream.
(3) From the viscera contained within the abdomen.
(4) Rarely through the diaphragm or by lymphatic extension from the thigh.

233

The only commonly blood-borne organism of importance is the pneumococcus, which may cause severe so-called primary peritonitis.

Organisms may reach the peritoneum from the contained viscera either by (*a*) rupture of a viscus or (*b*) by escape through the diseased wall of any viscus. In the female there is the additional path of infection via the Fallopian tube. Frequently a local abscess may form either extra- or intra-peritoneally near the diseased viscus, and later such abscess may burst into the general peritoneal cavity.

The common causes of general peritonitis are the conditions already described in previous chapters, and comprise disease or rupture of the hollow viscera, and ruptured abscess of the solid viscera.

> Perforation of the appendix vermiformis.
> Perforation of gastric or duodenal ulcer.
> Perforation of typhoid or tuberculous ulcer of small intestine.
> Perforation of dysenteric or stercoral ulcer or of a diverticulum of the colon.
> Perforation of gall-bladder, or biliary ducts.
> Gangrene of any strangled coil of gut, or intussusception, or volvulus.
> Infection spreading from a pyosalpinx.
> Infection spreading from an infected uterus.
> Infection spreading from a pyonephrosis.
> Rupture of a liver-abscess or splenic abscess.

The above comprise all the common causes of general peritonitis. The symptoms of peritonitis vary greatly according to the part and extent of the peritoneum involved, the nature of the infective agent, and the acuteness of onset. Help in diagnosis will be obtained by regarding the symptoms as being roughly grouped in two classes—reflex and toxic.

Pain.
Vomiting.
Anxious facial expression.
Rigidity of abdominal muscles. } Reflex.
Superficial hyperæsthesia.
Collapse. Alteration of temperature.

Distension. } Toxic
Intestinal paresis.
General toxæmia.

The importance in recognizing these two groups of symptoms lies in the facts that reflex symptoms are earlier in onset when a *demonstrative* part of the peritoneum is affected, but may be delayed considerably when a *non-demonstrative* part is affected. The division of the peritoneum into these two parts is based upon a relatively free or scanty cerebro-spinal nerve-supply. The anterior and lateral parts of the abdomen are lined by peritoneum well supplied by somatic nerves which bring about brisk reflexes. The pelvis and median portion of the posterior abdominal wall have a scanty cerebro-spinal supply, and in consequence irritation of these parts causes minimal reflex symptoms.[1]

Toxic symptoms are nearly always late in onset. There is indeed an inverse relationship between the two groups, since severe toxæmia diminishes the sensibility of the reflex arc. It thus follows that when a non-demonstrative part of the peritoneum (e.g. the pelvic) has been primarily affected

[1] See further details in Z. Cope's *Clinical Researches in Acute Abdominal Disease*, p. 21 *et seq.* (Oxford Medical Publications).

reflex symptoms may be minimal throughout, for oncoming toxæmia diminishes the reflexes from the demonstrative part as it becomes progressively involved. Unless this fact is appreciated it is easy to overlook a pelvic or central peritonitis until the infection has advanced to a serious extent.

It will be noticed that two symptoms—collapse and alteration of temperature—are included in both groups. Collapse, by which we mean obvious and rapid depreciation of the circulation and metabolism, may be seen either early or late in the course of peritonitis. In the early stage it is a reflex symptom, whilst later in the course of the disease it is the result of absorbed toxins. The early reflex collapse is usually quickly recovered from, though occasionally toxic collapse follows close on the heels of reflex collapse. Early collapse is absent in those cases which have an insidious onset and is less likely to occur when the silent area of peritoneum is primarily involved.

Alteration of temperature is common in peritonitis, but is not sufficiently constant or regular to be of much aid in diagnosis. Early collapse is accompanied by subnormal temperature, whilst the ingravescent stage of the disease is usually indicated by fever of an irregular type. In the later stages of peritonitis the temperature may be normal, subnormal, or slightly elevated.

The early and reflex symptoms of peritonitis may, in the absence of initial collapse, be extremely equivocal. They are more likely to be definite in young persons whose reflex arcs are normally more sensitive, and conversely they may be insignificant in old and debilitated patients.

Pain is the most constant symptom. It may be

confined to the local area of inflammation or
referred more generally over the abdomen. As the
peritonitis extends the pain-area also extends,
though the maximum pain is nearly always felt at
the initial focus. Tenderness is a constant feature
over any focus of peritoneal inflammation. Even
when rigidity is absent there is usually pain
felt on pressure over the affected site. Only twice
or three times have I seen this tenderness absent—
once or twice as the result of extreme toxæmia
dulling the sensorium, and once as the result of
extreme muscular rigidity which apparently prevented transmission of the applied pressure to the
underlying inflamed area.

Vomiting is common at the onset of peritonitis, but
is usually infrequent until late in the case. The
later vomiting is usually obstructive in character.

The change in *facial appearance*, though a guide
to the experienced, is something which cannot be
indicated satisfactorily in words. The white, drawn
face of initial collapse will tell anyone that something serious has happened, but collapse is by no
means constant. In any case, the reaction from
initial collapse is so rapid and complete that the
facial aspect commonly becomes and remains
almost normal for a time. But there is usually an
indefinable yet perfectly definite aspect of countenance in many persons who may present an otherwise doubtful picture of peritonitis. The Hippo-
cratic facies present in late peritonitis is merely
that of extreme collapse.

Muscular rigidity is a common accompaniment
of the early stages of peritonitis, *but only when the
part of peritoneum affected lies in the demonstrative*

area. It is best seen in perforation of a duodenal or gastric ulcer, whereby a large part of the demonstrative section of the peritoneum is irritated. It is generally absent or but slightly demonstrable when the peritonitis is limited to the pelvis. In those cases in which rigidity is present in the early stages the muscles relax as the peritonitis progresses, until in the final picture it is almost absent. Rigidity is also either absent or difficult to detect in fat people with flabby muscles and in old and weak patients. Rigidity may be of slight degree in some cases of pneumococcal peritonitis and in some of the slowly advancing infections due to the *bacillus coli* and streptococcus. When sterile bile or urine leaks into the peritoneal cavity the resulting irritation may not be accompanied by rigidity of the abdominal muscular wall. In cases of biliary extravasation several pints of bile may accumulate within the peritoneum before the increasing tumidity and distension, and the presence of free fluid within the abdomen reveal the serious nature of the condition.

Cutaneous hyperæsthesia is frequently seen in the subumbilical area of the abdomen in the region supplied by the tenth, eleventh and twelfth thoracic nerves. It is more frequently seen on the right side. Commonly it is limited to a narrow strip above each Poupart ligament.

The *toxic symptoms of peritonitis* are later in appearance and indicate a more serious stage of the disease. An occasional intermittence of the pulse is often one of the indications of advancing peritonitis. As the infection involves the various coils of intestine they become paralysed and distended, whilst the intestinal contents stagnate and increasing obstruction results. Poisonous substances are absorbed from the stagnating contents and secondary collapse results. At this stage true obstructive vomiting is commonly a feature, and there is noted the small running pulse commonly described as indicative of peritonitis. Such a pulse is felt in the *latest* stages of peritonitis, and not in the earlier stages when diagnosis is so important.

The differential diagnosis.—It is not difficult to diagnose a flagrant case of peritonitis, for the pain, vomiting, local tenderness, and muscular rigidity with fever sufficiently indicate the condition ; but mistakes are likely to be made either because the symptoms are too slight or because they are atypical. The early symptoms are slight and deceptive when the part primarily affected lies in the pelvis or in some other relatively silent area of the abdomen ; they are often atypical in patients who are old, debilitated, or very fat. In the late stages of peritonitis it is frequently impossible to differentiate from intestinal obstruction, which develops as a late consequence of peritonitis. We would take one more opportunity of emphasizing that the condition of the pulse is no true guide in diagnosing early peritonitis.

The conditions which may simulate peritonitis are:
    Pleuro-pneumonia.
    The colics.
    Intestinal obstruction.
    Internal hæmorrhage.
    Some nervous conditions, e.g. tabes, hysteria.

The differentiating points will be found enumerated in other parts of this book.

PRIMARY PNEUMOCOCCAL PERITONITIS

By primary pneumococcal peritonitis is meant that form of infection with the pneumococcus in which the peritoneal symptoms are the predominating feature of the illness. It is fairly reasonable to suppose that the peritoneal lesion is nearly always secondary to some other focus in the body, but when that focus is latent or of minor importance it is customary to use the above term.

Blood-infection without any ascertainable focus of origin does occur, but more frequently infection spreads from the Fallopian tube, or possibly from the intestine. The disease is much more common in females under the age of ten.

The symptoms vary considerably. They are those of peritonitis of varying grades of severity. One can with advantage describe three stages to the disease—the stage of onset, an intermediate stage, and a residual stage (Waugh).[1]

The **stage of onset** starts abruptly with abdominal pain, vomiting, and fever, which may reach 104° or 105° F. In some instances there is noticeable diarrhœa. Frequently there are toxic symptoms out of proportion to the local findings, and delirium may be noted.

The abdominal pain may be diffuse, but is usually more definite in the hypogastrium. The abdominal wall may be rigid, but more often is soft, and there may be but slight local tenderness.

In the very severe cases, which are always septicæmic for a time, death may occur within two or three days.

[1] See *Proc. Royal Soc. Med.*, 1924–5, voi. xviii, Dis. Children p. 51.

The **intermediate stage** corresponds to the formation of pus within the abdominal cavity. The toxic symptoms lessen, but irregular fever persists, and there is a gradual tumescence of the abdomen (Waugh). Leucocytosis will be observed. Abdominal pain in this stage is very slight, and the continued fever and a painless tumid abdomen may cause a suspicion of tuberculosis.

The **residual stage** corresponds to the definite localization of pus and the absence of all acute symptoms save fever of an irregular type. The pus may be in the pelvis, or in the central part of the abdomen, or even in the subphrenic region.

The *diagnosis* in the first stage has to be made from acute appendicitis. This is sometimes very difficult, but if the initial fever be high, if the abdominal signs are rather indefinite, and especially if there be slight delirium and troublesome diarrhœa, one should suspect pneumococcal peritonitis. The condition occurs chiefly in young girls, and some help may be obtained by examining the vaginal secretion for the pneumococcus, since Fraser showed that the Fallopian tube is the common route of infection. If there be any serious doubt it is wiser to recommend exploration, since more harm is likely to result from allowing a septic appendix to perforate than from exploring an early pneumococcal peritonitis.

In the intermediate stage the continued fever, tumidity of the abdomen, and comparative absence of abdominal pain and tenderness may lead to a suspicion of tuberculous peritonitis or even typhoid fever. The history of onset, the palpation of any enlarged glands or masses in the abdomen, or the positive result to a test for tuberculosis may help to diagnose the former; whilst the absence of leuco-cytosis, an enlarged spleen, and a positive agglutin-ation test would point to typhoid.

In the third or residual stage a definite swelling will be detected in some part of the abdomen ; this is a residual abscess, and may be in the pelvis or upper or middle abdomen. The diagnosis in this stage has to be made from the other causes of abdominal tumour and abscess. The history of the previous illness will be of the utmost importance in deciding on a diagnosis.

It has been mentioned above that pneumococcal peritonitis may not give rise to the muscular rigidity which is usual with most other forms of acute peritonitis. I have known the combination of abdominal pain, vomiting, and lax abdomen give grounds for diagnosing acute intestinal obstruction.

If there be coincident pleuritis or pericarditis the symptoms of peritonitis may be entirely over-shadowed. In the early stages of a pneumococcal polyserositis it is often very difficult to determine the exact diagnosis, but if definite signs declare themselves in the lung it would be inadvisable to recommend opening the abdomen until there are sufficient grounds for suspecting the presence of pus. If the thoracic condition has been success-fully treated, but the patient does not progress, special care must be paid to the abdomen, for the absence of rigidity and the comparatively slight pain may allow a considerable collection of pus to go unobserved. Waugh draws attention to the significant tumescence of the abdomen in these cases.

The prognosis in cases of pneumococcal peritonitis has been greatly altered for the better by the fact that the organism is sensitive to some of the antibiotics and the sulphonamide group of drugs. Early cases can be successfully treated by administration of penicillin and sulphadiazine, and thereby operation may be altogether avoided.

CHAPTER XIX

DISEASES WHICH MAY SIMULATE THE ACUTE ABDOMEN

THERE are a number of diseases which either do not need or positively contra-indicate operative interference, which may yet cause symptoms very suggestive of conditions for which operation is the best procedure. In some cases the symptoms arise from disease within the abdomen, in other instances the pain is referred to the abdomen from another part of the body, e.g. thorax or spine.

GENERAL DISEASES

It is not uncommon for abdominal pain and vomiting to occur at the onset of some of the specific fevers or of **influenza,** especially in children, but in such the general symptoms outweigh the local manifestations. Fever will be present at the start and the general malaise is greater, while locally there will not be found the tenderness or rigidity which suggest intra-abdominal inflammation, and it is by this discrepancy that the observer will be guided. Occasionally the abdominal symptoms may precede the general manifestations of influenza ; the pain may be of a severe colicky type, and if accompanied by vomiting may give rise to a suspicion of acute intestinal obstruction. The vomiting never tends to become fæculent and soon the general symptoms of influenza appear.

244

During an epidemic of influenza one is more likely to mistake an acute abdominal condition for a simple influenza with gastric symptoms—a serious mistake.

Diabetes.—Impending coma in diabetes is often accompanied by severe abdominal pain and vomiting. There may also be some rigidity and tenderness of the abdominal wall. The way is then clear for a misdiagnosis of acute inflammation within the abdomen and, indeed, mistakes of this nature have been made.

In order to avoid such mistakes the first step is the routine examination of the urine for sugar. If sugar is found the presence or absence of diacetic acid must be determined. If a ketosis is found the abdominal symptoms and signs must be very carefully observed and appraised. If there be any serious doubt about the diagnosis immediate steps should be taken to treat the ketosis by administration of insulin with glucose. If the abdominal symptoms are entirely due to diabetic condition they will very speedily subside under this treatment. If they do not show signs of subsiding the surgeon can be sure that there is a serious intra-abdominal condition present.

Typhoid fever is sometimes accompanied by abdominal pain and local tenderness, especially in the right iliac fossa (see Chapter V).

In tropical climes malaria frequently causes severe abdominal pain, but the type of fever and an examination of the blood easily enable one to diagnose.

Tuberculous peritonitis may cause vague abdominal pains, distension of the abdomen, and free

fluid.   These symptoms may occasionally give rise
to the opinion that there exists some acute abdominal condition.   The gradual onset of symptoms,
the tumidity of the abdomen, the lack of rigidity
and tenderness, and the presence of tubercle else-

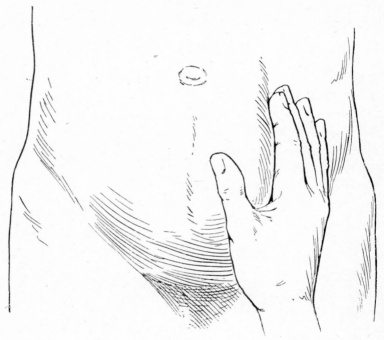

Fig. 39.—Diagram to show method of differentiating between right-
sided abdominal pain of thoracic and abdominal origin.   (Pressure
from the left side causes pain if abdominal in origin.)

where in the body may be sufficient to lead to the
correct diagnosis.

It must be remembered, however, that intestinal
obstruction and perforative peritonitis sometimes
occur in the course of tuberculous peritonitis, and
these demand operative treatment.   Sometimes
when the ileo-cæcal region is extensively involved

in the tuberculous process, the gut may be adherent in the iliac fossa and the simulation of appendicitis may be very close. There may also be superficial hyperæsthesia, but in acute tuberculous peritonitis this is usually more extensive than in appendicitis, reaching occasionally well above the umbilicus.

Food poisoning may give rise to abdominal pain, vomiting, and collapse. There is a serious pitfall here. Many patients who have a ruptured appendix or stomach attribute the trouble to the eating of some particular article of diet. One may therefore miss a condition needing surgical intervention, just as one may think an operation necessary when there is no need for interference. In food (or ptomaine) poisoning the symptoms usually follow definitely after eating some article of diet suspected to be tainted. Frequently several people are simultaneously attacked. In any case, though the general symptoms are similar, the local abdominal condition is unlike that of peritonitis (no rigidity) or severe obstruction (absence of fæculent vomiting), and there should usually be no difficulty in diagnosis if a careful watch be kept upon the case.

Bornholm disease or epidemic pleurodynia (epidemic myositis) sometimes has an onset which may cause it to be mistaken for an acute abdominal affection. The disease chiefly affects the muscles of the shoulder, chest and abdomen, which become painful. If the abdominal muscles are chiefly affected a cursory examination might lead one to suspect appendicitis, for there may be tenderness in the lower abdomen and superficial hyperæsthesia in the region of distribution of the 9th, 10th and 11th dorsal nerves. There is slight fever and often headache and nausea, sometimes diarrhœa. Differential diagnosis should not be difficult since the muscle-tenderness is found in the thoracic muscles also, and there is often pain on breathing and sometimes a pleuritic rub. Moreover, it is usual for several cases to occur about the same time.

BLOOD-DISEASES

The only blood-disease which I have ever known to cause simulation of acute abdominal disease is spleno-medullary leukæmia. The patient gave a history of prolonged indigestion, had suffered recently from irregular fever, and with an anæmic appearance presented also great tenderness, rigidity, and dullness in the left hypochondrium, so that the simulation of subphrenic abscess due to a leaking ulcer was rather close. A leucocyte count, however, showed 240,000 white cells to the cubic millimetre and the true condition was recognized. The acute local reaction was due to tension and threatening rupture of the spleen, for spontaneous rupture took place shortly afterwards.

Attacks of severe abdominal pain accompanied by vomiting (and sometimes diarrhœa) occur in some cases of pernicious anæmia, but seldom give rise to serious difficulty in diagnosis.

ACHOLURIC JAUNDICE

It is well known that this disease is sometimes accompanied by abdominal crises in which acute abdominal pain, nausea or vomiting, and tenderness on palpating the abdomen are noteworthy features. The attacks coincide with an increase in the depth of the jaundice and intensity of the anæmia. It is likely that these attacks are due to intra-abdominal hæmorrhage, and in the absence of other indications there is little need to open the abdomen. Removal of the spleen at a suitable time will free the patient from such attacks.

THORACIC DISEASES

Pleurisy or pleuro-pneumonia.—Either of these conditions may cause abdominal pain and rigidity, and may be accompanied by vomiting. In some cases it is quite easy to distinguish by the signs present in the chest, but in children in whom the thoracic signs are often late in appearing, and in some cases of diaphragmatic pleurisy in which few signs may be found, diagnosis is extremely difficult. I have discussed this subject more fully elsewhere,[1] but a summary of the main differential points will be found on p. 250.

An additional test is illustrated in Fig. 39. If the pain be unilateral and of abdominal origin pressure from the opposite side of the abdomen towards the affected side will cause pain, whilst if the pain be referred from the thorax no pain is caused by such pressure.

Acute cardiac disease frequently causes symptoms referable to the abdomen. Epigastric pain and tenderness are common when the liver is congested and swollen from back pressure; vomiting is not an infrequent symptom in cardiac failure, and severe collapse may usher in an attack of pericarditis or accompany acute cardiac failure. I have on occasion been called to cases of endocarditis, pericarditis,

---

[1] See *Clinical Researches in Acute Abdominal Disease* (Oxford Medical Publications).

COMPARATIVE TABLE OF SYMPTOMS IN ACUTE ABDOMINAL AND ACUTE PLEURAL OR PNEUMONIC LESIONS

ABDOMINAL.	PLEURAL OR PNEUMONIC.
Previous History— Indigestion. Colicky pains. Constipation. Diarrhœa.	Common cold or " chill." Exposure to infection.
Onset— Acute without fever (except pyelitis). Rigor unusual (except pyelitis). Vomiting usual. Pain often shifts downward.	Acute with fever at start. Rigor common. Vomiting less common. Pain thoracic as well as abdominal.

EXAMINATION.	
Appearance— Varies from normal to " abdominal " facies.	Cheeks flushed. Alæ nasi working. Sometimes herpes on lips.
Skin— Cold or clammy or normal.	Skin may be hot and dry.
Pulse and Respiration— No sure guide.	$\frac{P}{R}$ ratio lessened.
Abdominal wall— May be rigid.	Less commonly rigid.
Phrenic shoulder-pain— Common, but seldom below clavicle.	Common, especially below clavicle.
Skin hyperæsthesia— Common.	Rare, and never below level of navel.
Psoas test— Often positive.	Always negative.
Obturator test— Sometimes (rarely) positive.	Always negative.
Testicular pain— Sometimes present.	Never present.
Rectal examination— May elicit tenderness or demonstrate lump.	Negative.
Examination of chest— Frequently slight rubs in upper abdominal lesions.	May be a rub or dullness or bronchial-breathing, but sometimes nothing definite at onset of symptoms.

In cases which still remain doubtful after careful clinical examination, a small incision to the right of navel under morphine and local anæsthesia should be made.

and angina pectoris which were thought to be cases of abdominal disease. Needless to say, in any case of doubt, the circulatory system must be very carefully examined. It is indeed seldom that any doubt remains after one has measured the cardiac and hepatic dullnesses, listened to the cardiac sounds, noted carefully the character and rate of the pulse, and observed if there be any venous pulsation.

The only case in which I have known any reasonable doubt was that of a man of sixty to whom I was summoned in the middle of the night for a supposed perforation of a gastric ulcer. The patient had been under treatment for a twelvemonth for gastric ulcer which caused frequent attacks of indigestion. Sudden abdominal pain and collapse had supervened several hours before I was summoned. I found the patient fully conscious, very talkative, but extremely distressed and short of breath. No pulse could be felt at either wrist, nor could the brachial arteries be felt to pulsate. The heart was beating 160 to the minute, and the superficial veins of the neck were pulsating visibly. The liver was tender and enlarged down to the umbilicus. Pain was felt down the left arm to the elbow. I diagnosed cardiac failure and angina pectoris and refused to operate. The patient died five hours later, and a post-mortem examination of the abdominal cavity showed no gastric ulcer and no peritonitis. The thorax was not examined, but it was clear that the frequent attacks of indigestion had been slight attacks of angina pectoris. The diagnosis of cardiac failure would not have given rise to so much doubt if the gastric lesion had not been so confidently diagnosed previously.

Ordinary cardiac failure does not cause true rigidity of the abdominal wall, though pressure on a tender swollen liver may elicit muscular resistance. With acute pericarditis, however, there may be true rigidity of the abdominal wall, but this would be unaccompanied by other signs of abdominal disease. With pericarditis also there may be phrenic referred pain felt under the left clavicle. The significant pain down the left arm sometimes felt in cardiac disease may be helpful in diagnosis.

DISEASES OF THE SPINE OR SPINAL CORD

Acute osteomyelitis of the dorsal or lumbar *vertebræ* may cause abdominal pain and rigidity, but there will be great tenderness on pressure over the affected part of the spine which will draw attention to the origin of the pain.

In children acute abdominal (epigastric or umbilical) pain may be consequent on *Pott's disease of the spine*. The absence of abdominal signs would naturally cause examination of the spine and detection of the spinal disease.

Tabes dorsalis frequently causes severe abdominal pain in the form of *gastric crises*. The crises, though more common in adults, may also occur in children who are the subject of juvenile tabes. The pains may be very severe, and uncontrollable vomiting may occur. The important point to remember is that the abdominal wall is not rigid in the intervals of the pain of a gastric crisis.

When there is the slightest doubt about the diagnosis, it should be made a rule to test the pupillary reactions and the knee-jerks, so that the mistake will not be made of advising an abdomen to be opened when the pains are caused by tabes dorsalis. It must be recollected, however, that an acute abdomen may occur in a tabetic subject, and one should not hesitate to advise operation if the local signs are definite. A gastric crisis is most frequently mistaken for a perforated gastric ulcer, though careful examination should easily prevent this; a perforated ulcer has been sometimes misdiagnosed as a gastric crisis simply because the patient was found to be suffering from tabes dorsalis. It cannot be too strongly emphasized that persisting board-like rigidity of the abdominal wall indicates something more than a tabetic crisis.

RENAL DISEASE

Serious disease of the kidneys may cause uræmia, which may be accompanied by vomiting and abdominal distension. Thus intestinal obstruction may be closely simulated. This may occur either in acute nephritis, chronic nephritis, in bilateral cystic disease of the kidneys, or with pyonephrosis.

If in every case of intestinal obstruction one remembers the possibility of uræmia, there should be no great difficulty in diagnosis by considering the differential points set out below :

Intestinal obstruction.	Uræmia simulating obstruction.
Indication of renal failure absent.	May be very dry, furred tongue, and great thirst.
No albuminuria.	Albuminuria of variable amount.
Vomiting tends to become fæculent.	Vomiting not fæculent.
If obstruction low down, absolute constipation of flatus and fæces.	Bowels may return flatus after enema.

Intestinal obstruction.	Uræmia simulating obstruction.
May be history of subacute attack of obstruction.	May be history of some surgical or medical disease of kidneys.
No renal tumours.	In cystic disease bilateral renal tumours found.
Blood-pressure may be normal.	Blood-pressure likely to be much raised.

It is very seldom that the two conditions are confused when once the possibility of uræmia is considered.

RETRO-PERITONEAL CONDITIONS

When one considers that the majority of the early symptoms of peritonitis are reflex in character, and that the nerve-endings constituting the afferent part of the arc lie for the most part in the sub-peritoneal tissues, it is no wonder that various irritating lesions in the space behind the peritoneum may closely simulate peritonitis. Retro-peritoneal effusions, if considerable in amount, may also displace the large bowel and cause obstruction.

The chief lesions occurring in the retro-peritoneal tissues and liable to cause difficulty in diagnosis (apart from acute pancreatitis) are :

> Rupture of aneurysm of aorta or any of the big abdominal vessels.
> Dissecting aortic aneurysm.
> Retro-peritoneal hæmorrhage from injury of kidney, or spontaneous bleeding from renal growth.
> Retro-peritoneal extravasation of bile.
> Extravasation of urine into extra-peritoneal tissues from ruptured bladder, ureter, or pelvis of kidney.
> Pelvic subperitoneal infections.

In the early stages of many of these lesions it is extremely difficult, if not impossible, to diagnose with certainty from an intra-peritoneal lesion, but when a sufficient amount of blood, urine, or inflammatory fluid has collected in a part which can be examined diagnosis may be rendered more easy by a sign pointed out by Joyce. This sign, which is dependent upon the fact that a retro-peritoneal effusion is not movable, consists in a sharp line of demarcation between a dull fixed area and the resonant remainder of the abdomen ; it is of most value in perirenal extravasations, and in such cases the limiting line corresponds in position to the displaced ascending or descending colon, whilst the dull area occupies the loin and lateral part of the abdomen.

Retro-peritoneal extravasation of blood from rupture of an aneurysm of the abdominal aorta or one of the big abdominal vessels constitutes a grave emergency which can seldom be successfully treated by surgery. Diagnosis may be possible when the patient has been known to be suffering from an aneurysm. Sudden collapse and great abdominal pain would naturally direct one to the cause. In the absence of any previous history, diagnosis is often impossible. The sudden appearance of a painful retro-peritoneal swelling following collapse in a patient known to be suffering from severe arterio-sclerosis might make one suspect the rupture of an aneurysm. In a patient suffering from malignant endocarditis a mycotic aneurysm may form and rupture retro-peritoneally with the immediate appearance of a painful swelling and local rigidity of the abdominal wall. In one such case I made an erroneous diagnosis of perinephric abscess through not paying sufficient attention to the observation of a reliable observer that the swelling had not been there the night before I saw the patient.

Dissecting aneurysm may cause very severe abdominal pain, and occasionally local tenderness and rigidity of the abdominal wall. It is therefore easy to understand how it may rarely be mistaken for perforation of a peptic ulcer. With dissecting aneurysm, however, the collapse is extreme and more lasting, and the pain does not abate so soon as it does in the reactionary stage of a perforated ulcer ; moreover, the catastrophic pain always starts in the thorax and takes a few seconds to reach the abdomen. The local disturbance of blood-supply caused by a dissecting aneurysm may lead to a weak or absent pulse in one or other limb, and this may be associated with numbness and paræsthesia in the part affected. The absence of other characteristic signs of a perforated ulcer should easily serve to distinguish between the two conditions.

Severe mesenteric thrombosis causes symptoms very similar to those of dissecting aneurysm, and in the absence of a typical history I know no way of differentiating the two conditions.

Retro-peritoneal extravasation of bile is usually diagnosed only on opening the abdominal cavity. It causes symptoms of subacute peritonitis.

Pelvic subperitoneal infections, if acute, may cause some intra-peritoneal irritation. We have seen such symptoms caused by spreading gas-gangrene of the vulva, and Joyce[1] relates a case in

---

[1] See J. L. Joyce, *British Journal of Surgery*, vol. xii, No. 47, p. 547 *et seq.*

which severe abdominal symptoms followed on the mistaken injection of a soap-and-water enema into the perirectal tissues. In such cases there is some peritoneal irritation, the exact extent of which can often only be told by exploration.

INDEX